THE MAKING OF ADDICTION

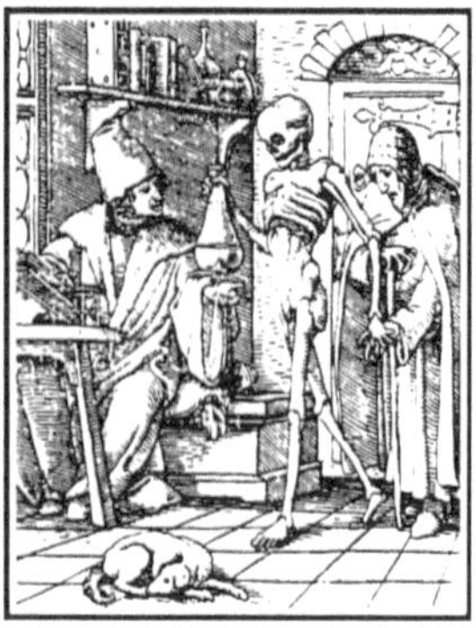

The History of Medicine in Context

Series Editors: Andrew Cunningham and Ole Peter Grell

Department of History and Philosophy of Science
University of Cambridge

Department of History
The Open University

Titles in this series include:

The Rise of Causal Concepts of Disease
Case Histories
K. Codell Carter

Florence Nightingale and the Health of the Raj
Jharna Gourlay

Health, Sickness, Medicine and the Friars in the Thirteenth and Fourteenth Centuries
Angela Montford

'The Battle for Health'
A Political History of the Socialist Medical Association, 1930–51
John Stewart

The Making of Addiction

The 'Use and Abuse' of Opium in Nineteenth-Century Britain

LOUISE FOXCROFT
Independent Scholar

Routledge
Taylor & Francis Group
LONDON AND NEW YORK

First published 2007 by Ashgate Publishing

Published 2016 by Routledge
2 Park Square, Milton Park, Abingdon, Oxon OX14 4RN
711 Third Avenue, New York, NY 10017, USA

Routledge is an imprint of the Taylor & Francis Group, an informa business

British Library Cataloguing in Publication Data
Foxcroft, Louise
The Making of Addiction: The 'Use and Abuse' of Opium in Nineteeth-Century Britain.
– (The History of Medicine in Context)
1. Opium abuse – Great Britain – History – 19th century. 2. Drug addiction –
Great Britain – History – 19th century. I.Title.
362.2'93'0941'09034

Library of Congress Cataloging-in-Publication Data
Foxcroft, Louise, 1956–
The Making of Addiction: The Use and Abuse of Opium in Nineteenth-Century Britain / Louise Foxcroft.
p. cm. – (The History of Medicine in Context)
Includes bibliographical references and index.
1. Opium – Therapeutic use – Great Britain – History – 19th century. 2. Opium abuse – Great Britain – History – 19th century. I. Title. II. Series.
RM666.06F69 2007
615'.323350941–dc22 2006016953

ISBN 9780754656333 (hbk)
ISBN 9781138275362 (pbk)

Contents

Part II: The Medical History of Addiction in Nineteenth-Century Britain

Acknowledgements

I owe my great thanks to Vic Gatrell whose advice on this book was indispensable and whose good humour scarcely failed him at all. The late Brian Outhwaite was unfailingly kind and encouraging, always generous with his time and patience. I am grateful, too, to Fiona Green who spent many hours discussing it all with me and then scrutinised the final draft. Any mistakes that remain are mine alone. My thanks, too, to Anna Abulafia for her constant support from the very beginning, and to Lucy Cavendish College, Cambridge for generously providing financial assistance.

But what is experience where opium is concerned?
Wilkie Collins, *The Moonstone* (1868)

Chapter One

Introduction

> The first dose is taken, and mark the transformation. This overmastering palliative creates such a confident, serene, and devil-may-care assurance that one does not for once think of the final result. The sweetness of such harmony can never give way to monotony. Volition is suspended … when distress supervenes, you go at once for the only balm that abounds in Gilead, and every additional dose is but another thread, however invisible, of which the web is made that binds us fast as fate.[1]

Perspectives on addiction

What does addiction mean to us now, what has it meant to others in the past, and how are all these meanings connected? The phenomenon of addiction has a long socio-cultural history but the field of knowledge that has developed around it is very recent. Historically, certain individuals have used 'certain substances in certain ways thought at certain times to be unacceptable by certain other individuals for reasons both certain and uncertain'.[2] But is this behaviour natural or pathological? Is it, even, morally reprehensible? This book is a social and intellectual history of the concept of addiction, concentrating on the use and abuse of opiates. It looks at public and personal perceptions of chronic opiate use in the nineteenth century and at the development of addiction as a medical condition, a disease entity, where, despite earlier experiences of 'habit' and 'enthralment', no such definition had previously existed. Contrary to Thomas De Quincey's dictum this thesis takes the opium-eater as its hero and not opium itself.[3]

The personal and imaginative life of the nineteenth-century chronic opium user could not help but fashion the medical and popular understanding of addiction. The experiences and ideas of opium users informed, influenced and manipulated medical knowledge in a cross-referential manner. Addiction was initially understood from a non-empirical, non-scientific viewpoint and even later, after the mid-nineteenth-century epistemological shift towards medicalisation of the condition, the concept was not based exclusively on pathological and physiological interpretation.

---

1 J.B. Mattison, 'Opium Addiction Among Medical Men', *Medical Record*, 1883, 23, pp.621-3.

2 H. Schaffer and M.E. Burglass, eds, *Classic Contributions in the Addictions* (1981), p.xix.

3 'Not the opium-eater, but the opium is the true hero of the tale', Thomas De Quincey, *Confessions of an English Opium Eater* (1821), p.78.

The disease entity of addiction was constructed from the 1860s onwards through the agency of medical experience; but in many respects this was too limited an experience, an accumulation of scientific knowledge and prejudice patched together in piecemeal fashion. Personal experience and medical theory were always interdependent but did not always coexist without controversy and conflict. For this reason the book is divided into two parts: the first, 'The Cultural History of Addiction in Nineteenth-Century Britain', explores the felt experiences of addicts and those around them, and the ways in which addiction was interpreted and presented; the second, 'The Medical History of Addiction in Nineteenth-Century Britain', traces the development of medical theory and practice.

Part I is a history of the many sorts of people who took the drug and became addicted to it, their reasons, needs, beliefs and sufferings for it, and the pleasure they found in it. Those who used opium, particularly for pleasurable or non-medical ends, have been largely ignored and yet their experiences add significantly to an understanding and history of addiction.[4] Chapter 2 focuses on the writings of Thomas De Quincey and Samuel Taylor Coleridge: their detailed and visceral experiences and explanations of addiction. Part I then goes on to look at the writings, letters and diaries of other opium users such as Elizabeth Barrett Browning, Lizzie Siddall, Dante Gabriel Rossetti, and Helen Gladstone, and at the responses of those who cared for, or were affected by, the opium user's habits. It looks at press and inquest reports that reveal everyday use; 'confessional' pieces, a popular genre which appeared in publications such as *London Society* and *Blackwood's Magazine*; articles on the Chinese opium dens of London which appeared under the cover of social investigation; and fictional descriptions in sensation novels employed as a melodramatic device. These are depictions that led a medical commentator in the 1870s to conclude that opiate use 'may indeed be said to have reached the height of fashion'.[5]

Why did people take opium? We might well ask ourselves why people do any of the things they do, and we could search for answers in an external scientific manner, empirically observing, measuring and interpreting behaviour, and also attending to personal accounts and explanations. It is attention to the latter which can best open up the history of addiction, and perhaps also give us valuable insight into the ways in which present-day theory and policy expose social norms, values and beliefs. Addiction as a medical condition or problem imposing a model of behaviour requiring treatment can then be seen as one more paradigm which can be deconstructed. It may be replaced with a 'process model' rather than the 'stochastic model' usually employed in pharmacological and psychological theories. The former is a 'dynamic process occurring over time, multifaceted in its origins, influenced by incidents and

---

4 For contemporary exposition of this argument see P. O'Malley and S. Mugford, 'The Demand for Intoxicating Commodities: Implications for the "War on Drugs"', *Social Justice*, 18, 4, pp.49-75.

5 Clifford Allbutt, 'On the abuse of hypodermic injections of morphia', *Practitioner*, 1870, 5, pp.327-31.

sequences that are pharmacological, psychological, historical, social, economical, political, [and] spiritual', whilst the latter implies an 'immutable process occurring in stereotypical fashion, not affected by change over time [where] historical and causal factors are unimportant'.[6] It is the pleasure that is experienced that defines what is now termed the 'motivational' factor in drug taking, and it is a history of use and pleasure that will redefine the basis of popular misconceptions common today. A greater understanding of this history would humanize the seemingly marginal figures who have used drugs in a non-medical way and dispel much of the demonisation which has attached itself to this behaviour.

The development of nineteenth-century medical opinion and treatment of addiction forms Part II of this book, since medicine was the most visible forum in which much of the debate took place. A protracted discussion of the nature of the newly designated 'disease', its aetiology, and the merits or otherwise of proposed therapies, took place in the second half of the nineteenth and early twentieth centuries. Although historians of opium have always referred to physicians and to their texts, no intensive account of this debate has yet been given. In the early nineteenth century the medical colonisation of opiates, which took place within the larger struggle of the profession for increased status, did not seriously vilify the 'luxurious' use of opium. By the end of the nineteenth century, however, the '*habitué*' was damningly diagnosed as suffering from a form of mental illness, and the treatment meted out to such persons was inextricably bound up in disease rhetoric as well as in prevailing theories of degeneracy and deviancy.

As the medical profession attempted to define addiction it unsurprisingly leant towards the iatrocentric, concentrating almost entirely on the physiological symptoms. Physicians noted, but did not accord any great significance to, the behavioural precursors and effects of an opium habit. By this means a schism of understanding was created between the physician and the user (assuming that they are in the main different creatures here, and for professional purposes they almost unfailingly were) and so allowed distrust and confusion, prejudice and fear, to arise around the condition. By the close of the century there was, broadly speaking, a parting of the ways resulting in two perspectives on perceived unorthodox drug use that would eventually be exacerbated by legislation in the first decades of the twentieth century. Neither approach could fully explain addiction and we might ask why one explanation came to be favoured over another and whether there was a 'danger of subordinating life to "science"', to the detriment of human well-being, inasmuch as the individual experience was marginalised.[7]

There are few recent historical works that include accounts of addiction, and, with the exception of Berridge and Edwards's *Opium and the People* (1981), they have all adhered largely unquestioningly to the idea of addiction as a 'given', a

6 J. Westermeyer, *Poppies, Pipes, and People* (1982), pp.60-1.

7 R. Richardson, *Death, Dissection, and the Destitute* (1988), p.xvii.

presupposed existing fact which was gradually uncovered and duly dealt with.[8] This persistent paradigm carries many misleading connotations and assumptions and it needs to be re-addressed. If it is, then addiction can be revealed as involving a known and ancient pattern of behaviour that gradually hardened into a recognised condition or disease entity, the latter emanating primarily from the animadversions of an increasingly cohesive and powerful medical profession.

This process, as I have suggested, has been generally treated in an unsatisfactorily linear and occasionally anachronistic fashion. Sonnedecker's essay, 'Emergence of the Concept of Opiate Addiction' (1962), for example, is whiggishly conservative, following the triumphant progress of the medical profession as it described and defined addiction. At the other end of the historiographic spectrum, Szasz, in his radical work *Ceremonial Chemistry: The ritual persecution of drugs, addicts and pushers* (1974), declared that there is no pharmacological basis to drug addiction and that 'in its present popular and professional use, the term "addiction" refers not to a disease but to a despised kind of deviance. Hence the term "addict" refers not to a bona fide patient but to a stigmatized identity, usually stamped on a person against his or her will'.[9] But there is an undeniable objective physiological reality to opiate addiction, differ as it may between individuals and environments, and these effects must also be recognised as contributing to the concept of addiction and to its stigmatization.

Szasz's challenging approach has, however, shifted away from the traditional arguments such as Sonnedecker's and, as Parssinen and Kerner have since suggested, the question is no longer, as Sonnedecker put it, 'how did medical men discover it?' but, following Szasz, 'why did they create it?'[10] Within the history and philosophy of science the evolution of scientific fact and the theory of paradigm change are mainly associated with the works of Fleck, Kuhn and Latour.[11] Accordingly, fact and theory develop and change as and when one set of principles and experimental practices are supplanted by others, and science then becomes whatever is generally accepted and acted upon by the scientific community at any given time.

---

8 See for example G. Sonnedecker, 'Emergence of the Concept of Opiate Addiction', *Journal Mondial De Pharmacie*, 1962, 3, pp.275-90; T. Parssinen, *Secret Passions, Secret Remedies: Narcotic Drugs in British Society, 1820-1930* (1983); G. Harding, *Opiate Addiction, Morality and Medicine* (1988); C.J. Acker, 'From all purpose anodyne to marker of deviance: physicians attitudes towards opiates in the U.S. from 1890 to 1940', in R. Porter and M. Teich, eds, *Drugs and Narcotics in History* (1995), pp.114-32.

9 T. Szasz, *Ceremonial Chemistry: The ritual persecution of drugs, addicts, and pushers* (1974), p.xv.

10 T. Parssinen and K. Kerner, 'Development of the Disease Model of Drug Addiction in Britain, 1870-1926' in *Medical History*, 1980, 24, pp.275-96.

11 The argument that scientific facts can be created and/or will evolve can be found in L. Fleck, *Genesis and Development of a Scientific Fact* (1935); T. Kuhn, *Structure of Scientific Revolutions* (1970); B. Latour, *Science in Action: How to follow scientists and engineers through society* (1987).

But a paradigmatic framework for analysis such as this can only be employed if it is assumed that addictive behaviour is explicable by scientific or quasi-scientific principles. Whilst the concept of addiction remains a subject for debate, the nineteenth-century medical profession did make this assumption. It treated addiction as an unnatural state and applied the reasoning of pathology to the problem in lieu of any other appropriate system of thought. As Latour suggests, 'uncertainty, people at work, decisions, competition, controversies are what one gets' when looking back at 'science in the making' and this dictum can be applied with some veracity to the medical construction of addiction in the nineteenth century.[12]

Berridge and Edwards alone have provided us with a thorough and impressive overview of Victorian consumption and attitudes to opium and its derivatives. But the 'nature and significance' of addiction is relegated to an appendix in the 1987 edition of *Opium and the People*. Here it is unequivocally stated that 'the opiates are drugs of addiction … anyone who takes an opiate for a long enough period and in sufficient dose will become addicted'. The main body of the work relies on this simplified basic premise and the nature and changing perspectives on addiction and on opium in the nineteenth century rest firmly upon it. This despite Berridge's statement in the 1981 edition of *Opium and the People* that, the 'vast outpouring of words on the "drug problem" … has produced no serious historical examination of the place of narcotics in English society'.[13] In the 1999 edition she states that 'concern about drug use has not quietened … but often the nature of understanding seems limited … contemporary definitions such as "addiction" … are transferred unthinkingly into the past'.[14] Little has changed; there is still a significant lack of secondary sources in English on the subject of the use and abuse of opiates in nineteenth-century Britain, and this pertains, too, to its wider international context.[15]

Further, it is argued that this 'problem' of opium use is a class issue, the 'outcome of the class bias of Victorian society', and it is thus understood as 'a question of social control'.[16] This assertion suggests a form of social plan or conspiracy perpetrated by certain interested parties in order to achieve a self-serving end. This is an argument I want to avoid. The medical theorisations of opiate use and the treatments that were

---

12 Latour, *Science in Action*, p.4.

13 Berridge and Edwards, *Opium*, (1981), p.xi.

14 Ibid. (1999), p.ix.

15 It is beyond the scope of this book to enter into the international debate, but contemporary American and European studies on addiction were to be found, reprinted or reviewed in the medical journals and often referred to in British medical texts. Oscar Jennings, for example, was not alone in referring to Levinstein's *Morbid Craving for Morphia (Die Morphiumsucht)*, published in London in 1878. Other studies familiar to nineteenth-century British physicians included: D.W. Cheever's article on 'Narcotics', first published in the *North American Review*, 1862, 95, pp.374-415; H. Day, *The Opium Habit: with suggestions as to the remedy* (NY, 1868); A. Calkins, *Opium and the Opium Appetite* (Philadelphia, 1871); H.H. Kane, *The Hypodermic Injection of Morphia. Its History, Advantages, and Dangers* (NY, 1880).

16 Berridge and Edwards, *Opium*, p.xxviii.

subsequently prescribed were less of a conspiracy than part of the unpredictable development of a scientific fact - of the uncertainties, controversies and decision-making described by Latour, which sprang from the overall 'rise of science' from the eighteenth century onwards. This is not to say that physicians and other professionals did not use some quite creative explanatory ideas to promote their own particular medical, material, political and philosophical interests, but it is why the debate needs to be looked at in greater depth.

Changing attitudes to drug addiction can be traced through successive editions of the *Oxford English Dictionary*. The first edition of 1897 defines the noun 'drug' as 'an original, simple medicinal substance, organic or inorganic, whether used by itself in its natural condition or prepared by art, or as an ingredient in a medicine or medicament'. What might be termed 'luxurious' use, indeed any description of use other than medicinal, does not receive any recognition until the publication in 1933 of the supplementary volume. There it is stated that the word 'drug' is 'now often applied without qualification to narcotics and opiates', and it is noted that the terms 'drug addict', 'drug evil', 'drug fiend', and 'drug habit' are commonly associated with this usage. Similarly in the *Index Medicus*, established in 1879 as a worldwide guide to medical periodical literature, 'Alcoholism' is the only cause of what can be termed 'substance abuse' mentioned in the first four volumes. In the fifth volume, however, published in 1883, this section had become 'Alcoholism, Opium Habit etc.'[17] Language and shades of meaning, as we shall see, are far from innocent representations of condition. They might be said to construct as well as reflect understanding.

Modern definitions of addiction

Whilst it would be misleading and anachronistic to apply modern drug addiction theories retrospectively, it is useful to look at this body of knowledge and to explain it in brief, plain terms, the better to understand where it has come from. Many people today share a simplistic picture of what drug addiction is and what it can do to an individual, any individual. Joseph Segen, in *Current Medical Talk: A Dictionary of Medical Terms, Slang and Jargon* (1995), gives a definition of addiction in layman's terms as 'a physiologic, physical or psychological state of dependency on a substance, which is characterised by tolerance, and a withdrawal syndrome when intake of the substance is reduced or stopped'. Taking his cue from World Health Organisation [WHO] deliberations he cites the defining elements as:

- Taking the drug more often or in larger amounts than intended
- Unsuccessful attempts to quit, persistent desire to use the agent, craving for the drug
- Excessive time spent in procuring the drug

17 J. Parascandola, 'The Drug Habit: The association of the word "drug" with abuse in American history', in Porter and Teich, *Drugs and Narcotics*, pp.156-67.

- Intoxication or withdrawal symptoms at inappropriate times
- Sacrifice of other activities or things for the drug
- Continual use of the drug despite knowledge of its harm
- Marked tolerance for the drug
- Typical withdrawal symptoms
- Use of drug to avoid or alleviate withdrawal symptoms.[18]

According to the WHO a drug is any substance which when taken into the living organism may modify one of its functions.[19] Modern popular views of opiates are that they are a powerful and supremely addictive family of drugs and that they induce feelings of great pleasure but at a dreadful physical cost if withdrawn. It is generally considered that the detrimental effects of chronic drug use on an individual are so obvious that they need no elucidation. In 1962, for example, the United States Supreme Court expressed this prevailing popular view in arguing that:

> to be a confirmed drug addict is to be one of the walking dead … the teeth have rotted out, the appetite is lost, and the stomach and intestines don't function properly. The gall bladder becomes inflamed; eyes and skin turn bilious yellow … good traits of character disappear and bad ones emerge. Sex organs become affected. Veins collapse and livid purplish scars remain. Boils and abscesses plague the skin; gnawing pain racks the body. Nerves snap; vicious twitching develops. Imaginary and fantastic fears blight the mind and sometimes complete insanity results. Often times, too, death comes much too early in life … Such is the torment of being a drug addict; such is the plague of being one of the walking dead.[20]

Addiction is still widely believed to be a universally destructive behavioural trait warranting a powerful response. But the persistence of opiate use, as a remedy and as a luxurious euphoric for over 6,000 years, raises many questions about the possibility of eradicating its unorthodox use. Addiction is a complex concept and many of the generally accepted assumptions about it, noted above, have been contradicted by more recent medical and sociological findings. These stress that drugs do not always do the same things to the same individuals, let alone to different people, and that the effects are due less to the intrinsic nature of the substance than to the situations in which the drug taking occurs. There now exist many studies that have failed to find scientific evidence that the habitual use of opiates causes 'chronic psychosis or an organic type of degeneration'. Indeed, it could be said that by far the most harmful effects of being a modern addict are due to the narcotics laws, and that any somatic or psychological illnesses are more likely to be due to adulterants and environment than to the drug itself.[21] Some now argue that the effects of drugs, including addicted

---

18 J. Segen, *Current Medical Talk: A Dictionary of Medical Terms, Slang, and Jargon* (1995), p.12.

19 T. Silverstone and P. Turner, *Drug Treatment in Psychiatry* (1978), p.3.

20 E.M. Brecher, 'Effects of opium, morphine, and heroin on addicts', *The Consumers Union Report on Licit and Illicit Drugs* (1972), p.92.

21 Ibid.

states, can often be seen as determined initially by the environment in which drug use occurs and then by the way the individual responds to it. If this is so then a purely substance or physiologically oriented understanding of what addiction is will be 'undermined by important considerations of the psychological (set) and the social (setting) environment in which it occurs'.[22]

Just as the effects of drugs have been found to be extraordinarily complex, so has the understanding of the concept of addiction. It has usually been seen as the result of the compelling properties of the drug itself or as a disease entity, either of the body or of the will, or both. If, though, it is something that is as much 'learned (and by this is meant culturally determined), as it is pathological (and so can be produced), then the given nature of addiction can be questioned. We may be able, as a result, to understand more about the structures of thought and the cultural restraints of a particular society which flow around a drug, as well as the nature and reality of individual experience. Addiction could then be seen as not only occurring where substances are involved but as just one element in a broader concept which would also account for a range of other 'addictive behaviours' such as compulsive and excessive gambling, eating, sexual activity, etc. If, as has been suggested, addictive behaviour is learned as well as pathological then perhaps it can be unlearned. If it is an 'impression on the soul' perhaps that impression can be lifted.[23] Understanding the history of addiction may involve questions of semantics, shades of meaning, rather than, or as much as, it involves an accumulation or interpretation of scientific knowledge.

This sort of conceptual understanding of drug addiction would need to give greater weight to the social and cultural elements that are involved in behaviour and definition, and which become something more than occasional and non-problematic. Biology and pharmacology would be given less significance and the 'given' nature of addiction, as something which simply exists and that we merely need to know more about to understand, could be questioned.

Opium in context: a brief history of antiquity of use, methods of production, and means of imbibing it

Opium is extracted from the poppy, botanically classified as *Papaver somniferum*, the genus being named from the Greek for poppy and the species from the Latin term for 'sleep inducing'. John Jones MD, writing in 1700 and one of the earliest British physicians investigating the drug, described raw opium as a 'most turgid of *Milky Juice*' which bleeds from the unripe seed pod of the flower when it is slit with a blade. The process required some care:

---

22 For a more comprehensive discussion of these ideas see R. Miller, 'What drugs do to users', in R. Coomber, ed., *Drugs and Drug Use in Society* (1994), pp.5-23; J.L. Falk, 'Drug dependence: myth or motive?', in Coomber, ibid., pp.44-57.

23 Thomas Trotter, *Essay, Medical, Philosophical, and Chemical, on Drunkenness* (1804), p.133.

> several incisions [are made] transversely or *athwart* the Head of the *Poppies*, yet not directly *horizontal*, but somewhat *obliquely* ... *They did not* make the *incisions quite through*, (if they could avoid it) lest any of the *Juice* should run through into the *Cavity* of the *Head*, and so be lost among the *Seeds* contain'd therein.[24]

Opium had already been known and used for some six thousand years and is referred to in Sumerian ideograms dating from c.4000 BC where the poppy is referred to as the 'plant of joy'. It is noted in Asyrian medical tablets of the seventh century BC, and in Mesopotamian, Egyptian and Persian texts from the second century BC. It occurs in fragments of veterinary and gynaecological papyri and in the Therapeutic Papyrus of Thebes of 1552 BC, and is described by Theophrastus and Dioscorides in the *Materia Medica* as having pain-killing and sleep-inducing properties. Helen's drug 'nepenthe', described in Homer's *Odyssey*, which brought 'forgetfulness of evil' and dissolved the grief of the Trojan Wars as well as that of the death of Ulysses, is thought to have been opium mixed with wine. Such a preparation was probably also used by initiates of the cult of Demeter, the goddess who, whilst searching for her lost daughter Persephone, came to Sicyon once known as Mecone, city of poppies, and on tasting opium forgot all her sorrows.[25]

The doctor-priests of Aesculapeius are thought to have treated the sick with opium, allowing them to sleep in sanctuary to experience a divinely inspired healing dream. Virgil mentions it as a soporific in the *Aeneiad* and in the *Georgics*. The Romans acquired knowledge of opium from the Greeks, and the surviving texts of Galen, the second-century physician and advocate of the drug, influenced European medical knowledge for many centuries. Following the decline of the Roman Empire its use spread to the Middle East, whence Arab traders carried it into Persia, India, China, Egypt, North Africa and Spain. During the Mohammedan conquest of the tenth and eleventh centuries the opium trade came to be established in Europe. John Arderne, writing in England in the fourteenth century, recommended opium as a soporific and as an external anaesthetic that the patient 'schal slepe so that he schal fele no kuttyng', and the iconoclastic Swiss physician Paracelsus (1490-1540) owed much of his following to the administration of opium, his 'stone of immortality'. Paracelsus was the first to use the term 'laudanum', but it was the seventeenth-century 'English Hippocrates', Thomas Sydenham, later known as 'Opiophilos', who gave the people laudanum as an alcoholic tincture and who broke out in 'praise of the great God, the giver of all good things, who hath granted [opium] to the human race, as a comfort in their afflictions'.[26]

The opaque, viscous liquid, bled from the poppy pod, is hardened to become a sticky, dark brown, pungent smelling stuff which is then scraped from the plant and smoked or swallowed, or put through various refining processes which serve to concentrate the active ingredients of the drug. These are the alkaloids that

---

24 John Jones, *The Mysteries of Opium Reveal'd* (1700), p.1.

25 J. Scarborough, 'The opium poppy in Hellenistic and Roman medicine', in Porter and Teich, *Drugs and Narcotics*, pp.4-23.

26 Ibid.

characteristically contain nitrogen and have a particularly bitter taste. More than fifty such compounds have been identified in crude opium latex, including noscapine, papaverine, codeine, thebaine, and morphine, the major constituent, which might average up to 20 per cent.[27] A toxic dose of opium must be ten times larger than an equivalence of morphine for fatal effects. Raw opium's analgesic action results generally from its morphine which acts directly as a depressant on the thalamus, the sensory cortex, and the respiratory and cough centres, but other alkaloids (especially those already mentioned) have stimulant action on the medulla and the spinal cord: papaverine and noscapine, in particular, relax intestinal muscle, thereby providing a modern explanation of the use of raw opium in the treatment of digestive disorders since antiquity. The pharmacist Friedrich Wilhelm Sertürner isolated morphine from raw opium in Hanover in 1807, naming it after Morpheus the Greek god of dreams, and published his classic paper on the drug in 1817. Heroin, a semi-synthetic opiate, was derived from morphine in 1874 at St Mary's Hospital in London by modifying the chemical structure of the natural substance. It was rediscovered in Germany in the 1890s and marketed by Bayer under the trade name of Heroin, taken from the German 'heroisch' meaning large or powerful in medical terminology.

However, it was raw opium that was most widely and freely resorted to for much of this period. The ways in which one could take opium changed very little if at all over the centuries; it was either swallowed in small rolled pills, or in the tincture of alcohol known as 'laudanum'. The latter, a draught that was ubiquitous by the mid-nineteenth century, was available at a cost of around one penny for twenty or twenty-five drops.[28] The drug also became increasingly available, for people of all ages, in any number of popular proprietary medicines such as 'Godfrey's Cordial', 'Black Drop', 'Dovers Powders', and 'Battley's Syrup'. Less frequently but more notoriously it was indulged in by smokers, with an astonishing amount of special drug paraphernalia. The following account from 1868 reveals that a small common oil lamp was brought out:

> lit and placed in the centre of a piece of cloth. Next [was] produced a small box containing his smoking tools, and finally a little gallipot and an instrument like a flute, with a wooden cup with a lid screwed on it at a distance of about three inches from the end. It was not a flute, however, but a pipe ... It was simply an eighteen-inch length of yellow bamboo with the cup of dark-coloured baked clay before mentioned fitted into a sort of spiggot hole near the end ... The stuff in the gallipot looked exactly like thin treacle, and smelt like burnt sugar and laudanum ... it had yet to be cooked - grilled. Taking an iron bodkin from his little tool chest [he] dipped the tip of it into the semi-liquid stuff, and withdrawing a little drop of it, held it in the flame of the lamp until it hardened somewhat. Keeping this

---

27 Crude opium contains morphine (up to 20%), noscapine (up to 8%), codeine (up to 2.5%), papaverine (up to 2.5%), thebaine (up to 2%), and smaller amounts of narceine, protopine, hydrocotarnine, and the other alkaloids, as well as meconic acid (the fifty alkaloids are largely combined with this organic acid) and some lactic and sulfuric acid among other constituents including up to 25% water.

28 See Appendix 1 for strengths and doses.

> still on the point of the bodkin, he dipped it again into the gallipot and again held it in the lamp flame, and repeated the process until a piece the size of a large pea was accumulated and properly toasted. This was placed in the pipe bowl ... It was lit at the little lamp [and the smoker] took the pipe-stem in his mouth. There is no mouthpiece to the pipe; the stem is cut sheer off, leaving something as thick as an office ruler to suck at ... there was at once emitted from the pipe a gurgling sound ... As the smoker ... sucked harder, swallowing all the black smoke except just so little as he was bound to waste in the process of breathing. He was as economical as could be, however, and expelled but the merest thread of the precious smoke through his nostrils and none by means of his mouth.[29]

There were no restrictions on opium use until the first Pharmacy Act of 1868. Due to long-running internal disagreements and struggles for status within the medical profession, the Act merely required that opium be labelled as a poison and free availability continued at the discretion of the individual druggist. Ironically, professional wrangling had prevented effective control as early as 1757 when a Bill was presented to the House of Commons calling for the powers to '*Restrain and Limit the Vending and Disposing of Poisons*'. The aim of this legislation had been to protect the status and business of apothecaries and chemists and, in so doing, prevent 'the mischievous Effects which may happen by the easy procuring of Drugs, and Chymical and Galenical Compositions or Preparations, of a poisonous Nature or Quality'.[30] It must be remembered that the drug was primarily used as a painkiller and sedative. It was the only effective analgesic available at that time to people living with poor sanitation, pathogenic environments, and limited access to often rudimentary medical care. Aspirin, for example, now similarly and routinely self-administered, was not introduced to the market until 1899.

Drugs had traditionally been sold by an eclectic group of traders including apothecaries, tailors, bakers and rent collectors. In the 1850s the number of people engaged in selling opium was estimated to be between 16,000 and 26,000, perhaps a conservative guess. The raw opium was often prepared in a shop with penny portions cut from a one-pound block and wrapped in packets. Many shopkeepers also sold their own opium preparations and there was an ever present and much commented on danger of accidental poisoning and overdose.[31] According to the author of a report in the *Edinburgh Medical and Surgical Journal* in 1808, Godfrey's Cordial contained a quarter of a grain of opium 'in each ounce of the liquid', and 'it is a fact, that this poison is sold … under three or four different proportions, one with twice the quantity of opium to another'. This, it was suggested, accounted for the level of infant mortality through accidental poisoning.[32] That there was general anxiety about growing home consumption and illicit use was revealed in a report in the *Times* on

29 Anon., 'East London Opium Smokers', *London Society*, 1868, 14, pp.68-72.

30 S. Lambert, *House of Commons Sessional Papers* (1975), 10, pp.219-26.

31 Berridge and Edwards, *Opium,* pp.24-7.

32 *Edinburgh Medical and Surgical Journal*, 1808, 4, pp. 271-2. There were many such cases of accidental poisonings of children, see for example 'Poisoning of an Infant by Syrup of Poppies', *Lancet*, 1858, 2, p.7.

8 March 1852. It related and discussed the annual accounts of 'trade and navigation' stating that the:

> quantity of opium entered for home consumption in 1850 amounted to 42,324 lb., and during the past year it had increased to 50,368 lb., being an increase of 8,044 lb. over that of the previous year, and a considerable increase of that of preceding years ... It would, therefore, appear that there is some truth in the report that … opium eating increases.[33]

Much of the opium on sale in Britain throughout most of our period did not originate in either India or China, as might be expected from British involvement in the opium wars of 1839-42 and 1856-58, but from Turkey, a source which captured over 70 per cent of the market even at the end of the century.[34] It arrived at several British ports but London's Mincing Lane saw the bulk of the dealing, in both open auction and private arrangements, involving opium brokers and large London wholesale drug houses such as Allen and Hanbury's and the Apothecaries' Company. Some of these bodies had been in existence since the seventeenth century. According to Berridge's calculations, per capita imports of opium entered for home consumption increased from an annual average of 1.62 lbs per 1,000 population in the period 1827-31 to 2.89 lbs in the years 1856-60, but it is difficult to know whether home consumption continued to rise after 1860 when duty on opium was eliminated. Berridge's estimated figures, which show great variation over time, have drawn decisive criticism and uncertainty remains.[35]

Concluding remarks

This book draws together the many and diverse threads that fed the mid-nineteenth-century epistemological shift in thinking and approaches to narcotics addiction. Today it is still argued that addiction is 'rooted in a multitude of disciplines', not only in medicine, psychology, physiology, and pharmacology, but also in 'history, sociology … philosophy, politics, witchcraft and religion to name but a few'.[36] A crisis of categories existed within the body of knowledge associated with addiction then as it does now. It has recently been suggested that there is a 'lack of integration between theory, research and practice', and that there is a 'failure to successfully coordinate the solution of scientific, technical and practical problems'.[37] Theorists and practitioners still debate the necessity, efficacy, rationality and even the morality of treating addictive behaviour, arguing, for example, over the relative merits of

33 *Times*, 8 March 1852, p.2, col.e.

34 Indian opium was occasionally found on the English market and it increasingly came from Persia too. There were even largely unsuccessful small-scale attempts at domestic cultivation. See Berridge and Edwards, *Opium*, pp.4, 11.

35 See T. Parssinen's Essay Review of Berridge and Edwards, *Opium*, in *Medical History*, 1982, pp.458-62.

36 Schaffer and Burglass, *Classic Contributions*, p.481.

37 Ibid., pp.xxxix, 483.

the substitution of alternative drugs such as methodone, and the recommendation of absolute abstinence instead of treatment for a possible underlying disorder or problem. If there existed across the nineteenth century an ambivalent and multi-faceted understanding of addiction and opium use, then it remains with us today.

PART I
The Cultural History of Addiction in Nineteenth-Century Britain

Chapter Two

The Experience of Addiction in the Early Nineteenth Century

> *Historian! You who celebrate bygones!*
> *You have explored the outward, the surface of the races – the life that has exhibited itself,*
> *You have treated man as the creature of politics, aggregates, rulers, and priests;*
> *But now I also, arriving, contribute something ...*
> *I press the pulse of life that has hitherto seldom exhibited itself, but has generally sought concealment,*
> *I illuminate feelings, faults, yearnings, hopes.*
>
> Walt Whitman, *Leaves of Grass* (1860-61)

Experience and empathy

To enliven an understanding of Victorian ideas and experience of addiction we need to look at the history of imagination and feeling as well as of medicine, to recognise the influence of reason and also, perhaps, of unreason. Such an approach is not a trivialisation of the subject, and particularly not of this one, where so much of the hidden material took place in the mind. Giving meaning to the idea of addiction, beyond that articulated merely in the physician's professional and material interests, allows us to see the scientific interpretation as lacking in, or unable adequately to convey, the imaginative experience or even the freedom of thought that arose from indulgence and which could provide a route to empathetic resonance. It is a very difficult thing to articulate a sense of wonder or terror, or even ennui, in scientific language alone.

The 'fascinating spectacle' of the nineteenth century 'struggling for inwardness' through intimately confessional diaries and letters, biographies and autobiographies, novels, self-portraits and histories has been elucidated by Peter Gay in volume four of *The Bourgeois Experience: Victoria to Freud* (1995). The 'self' that awaited either discovery or invention was, depending on the nature of the explorer, a subjective or an objective entity, either idealist or materialist, and sometimes both. Gay uses Freud's theory of mind, that the self is a part of nature, organised and as subject to causality as any physical form, and argues that 'any expression, no matter how banal or absurd – a dream, a fantasy, a slip of the tongue, a symptom, a linguistic habit', is a valid source for the historian.[1]

The human self, according to Freud and to Gay, is moulded by 'ideals and fears, incentives and threats', as well as 'instinctual urges'. It is an 'organism in conflict', labouring under competing and demanding appetites which vie for supremacy and are usually at odds with the needs of civilisation. Acknowledging that the application of Freudian theory is less than popular with most historians, Gay nonetheless asserts that they are all psychologists depending 'for the most part on prosaic generalisations about human behaviour', which, whilst they go some way to interpreting historic figures, fall short of a deeper understanding of inner life.[2]

As a tool for historians psychoanalytical psychology is controversial and contentious but it can also be fortuitously revealing of that 'deeper understanding'.[3] To apply it is not to be anachronistic if it is used to interpret material, as opposed to informing or dictating it, as it was in the later nineteenth century. 'Psychology' at that time did not refer to an established science but to a wide variety of topics concerning mental life that engaged the attention of educated people. Referring to the study of the soul, the term was known on the Continent in the mid-seventeenth century, and was used by David Hartley in his *Observations on Man* (1749). But it was unclear whether this new 'science of the mind' would be an empirically based analytical scheme or whether it would be conceptual and infinitely speculative. Would it follow the traditional route of experience, experimentation and observation or would it necessarily have to rely on subjective knowledge and introspection alone?

It has been argued that the 'powerful sense of the importance of the non-rationality of the depths and privacy of the human self', a sense that was such a

1 P. Gay, *Naked Heart* (1995), p.8.

2 Ibid., pp.9-10.

3 Psychohistory is a controversial tool for the historian, though it has established precedents: R.G. Collingwood, in his work *The Idea of History* (1956), stated that history is about past actions that lead to human self-knowledge; it is the explanation of motive and meaning. Peter Gay argues, in *Freud for Historians* (1985), that it is an informed style of inquiry, supplying answers no one had thought were available before, and, more importantly, suggesting questions no one had yet thought to ask. Controversy arises where, as Gay describes it, the historian takes a rapid tour through the tenets of psychoanalysis without a compass and ignorant of the language. I want to suggest that a psychohistorical approach could be useful when reading personal accounts of addiction, such as De Quincey's and Coleridge's, though wanting to avoid Gay's stated pitfalls, I have not undertaken this myself. Suggested texts for further reading include: Peter Gay, *Freud for Historians* (1985); Lloyd DeMause, *Foundations of Psychohistory* (1982); Jacques Szaluta, *Psychohistory: Theory and Practice* (1999); and for further reference Henry Lawton's *The Psychohistorian's Handbook* (1988). John Barrell's *The Infection of Thomas De Quincey. A Psychopathology of Imperialism* (1991) concentrates on questions of subjectivity raised by De Quincey's writings, but in the context of the early nineteenth-century concern with the nature and development of empire, rather than with that writer's experience of addiction. Nonetheless, it offers a psychopathological approach to De Quincey's body of work which illuminates the '*co-operation* of [his] internal and external terrors'.

distinctive contribution of the Romantic period, was neither successfully examined nor plausibly explained by physicians. It became instead the province of writers of fiction and poetry. This growth of interest is apparent in the works of such as De Quincey: in the 'strange, bizarre, mysterious, or unconscious aspects of mental life, and also in the emphasis that should be given to the unique character of each person'.[4] Many of those associated with Romanticism, a collective term for theories of art, of the imagination, and of language, applied posthumously, as it were, in the 1860s, were also at the cutting edge of medical and scientific knowledge.[5] Given this provenance, an inquiry into the parallax nature of attitudes to opium should begin with the recorded experiences of those who had explored the internal self and the external scientific.

Thomas De Quincey and the experience of addiction

It would be foolish to embark upon an exploration of the personal experiences of the nineteenth-century chronic opium user without acknowledging the centrality of Thomas De Quincey, and of the genre of confessional work, despite the extensive enquiries that have already been devoted to the man and his writing in many notable studies.[6] With bleak astonishment at his own servility and that of others, he had asked the rhetorical question: 'How came any reasonable being to subject himself to such a yoke of misery, voluntarily to incur a captivity so servile, and knowingly to fetter himself with such a seven-fold chain?'[7] He could not have been the first to ask himself this question. Many men and women had been held captive by opium before him and, whilst their individual stories were unique, they could not but conform in their shared experience of this slavery.

The *Confessions of an English Opium-Eater* was written in a series of opium-induced 'artificial respites' from illness and melancholia during the autumn of 1821. It was published in *The London Magazine* for October and November of that year, bringing the author the 'magnificent' sum of forty guineas, almost universal praise, and lasting fame and infamy. Horace Smith, author of *Rejected Addresses*, declared there was 'nothing so original and interesting in periodical literature'. Charles Knight wrote in the *Guardian* that the work had 'all the circumstantial sincerity of

---

4 R. Brown, 'Psychology', in I. McCalman, ed., *An Oxford Companion to The Romantic Age: British Culture 1776-1832* (1999), pp.361-9.

5 M. Butler, *Romantics, Rebels and Reactionaries: English Literature and its Background 1760-1830* (1981), p.1; R. Porter, 'Medicine', in McCalman, *Oxford Companion to The Romantic Age*, pp.170-7; N. Vickers, *Coleridge and the Doctors 1795-1806* (2004), passim.

6 See for example Hayter, *Opium and the Romantic Imagination*; G. Lindop, *The Opium-Eater: A Life of Thomas De Quincey* (1981); M. Elwin, *De Quincey* (1972); A.H. Japp, *Thomas de Quincey: His Life and Writings* (1890).

7 De Quincey, *Confessions*, p.4.

Defoe', though whilst praising the piece he also questioned its veracity.[8] The work was sufficiently notorious to merit several parodies, such as that which appeared in *Blackwood's Magazine* in 1823 under the title 'Confessions of an English Glutton'.[9]

De Quincey regarded his confessions as seminal and definitive. He had written 'the doctrine of the true church on the subject of opium'.[10] Describing the work thus, he was attempting to infuse it not only with all the liturgical *gravitas* of established religious reverence and supplication but also with the implicit, perhaps ironic, idea of the Christian *habit* of worship. He was suggesting to his readers that worshipping opium, giving oneself over to it, was analogous with a legitimate form of faith and religious indulgence. It was a Eutychian experience: human nature was merged with the divine. Opium was given its iconoclastic status by the highest authority, echoing the sixteenth-century physician Thomas Sydenham's claims that it was nothing less than a gift of God. In this mythical 'true church' De Quincey occupied the self-appointed roles, firstly, of a disciple in the 1821 edition, then as a noviciate and, thirty-five years later, as a Pope incarnate, so becoming, in his own words, 'consequently infallible'.[11] His metaphorical creed encompassed paradise, suffering, celestial visions, and, should it ever have attained earthly form, would have had 'altars and priests consecrated to its benign and tutelary powers'.[12] This church had many 'poor opium-martyrs' too, appropriate to an outlawed and unorthodox creed, amongst whose ranks he suggested the inclusion of Samuel Taylor Coleridge, a seraphic wastrel, a 'damaged archangel'.[13] Martyrdom to opium in these terms was laudable if not glorious; it set the user apart from, singled out and above his fellows, and also at a magnificent distance from the later medical model of a reviled pathological degenerate.

---

8 Elwin, *De Quincey*, pp.98-9. The opium-eater was suddenly a literary sensation and at a dinner given in his honour by the publishers he was fêted by Lamb, Hazlitt, Thomas Hood and, among others, Thomas Griffiths Wainewright. The latter was better known to the public by his *London Magazine* pseudonym, 'Janus Weathercock', and, infamously, he was later transported for murder by poisoning; see A. Motion, *Wainewright the Poisoner: The Confessions of Thomas Griffiths Wainewright* (2000).

9 S.M. Levine, *The Romantic Art of Confession* (1998), p.25. When *The London Magazine* published the first installment of the *Confessions* it sold 1,700 copies but the parodic articles in *Blackwood's Magazine* reached a far greater audience, typically c.14,000, thus a far larger readership was introduced to De Quincey's work.

10 De Quincey, *Confessions*, p.42.

11 Ibid. (1821), p.42; (1856), p.265.

12 Ibid.; Hayter, *Opium and the Romantic Imagination*, p.104. Hayter refers to De Quincey's use of religious imagery and language as a 'disagreeable practice', arguing that it is 'miserably true' that he inspired others' curiosity in opium which led inexorably to their addiction. Such arguments can be heard still from those who maintain that ignorance acts as a safeguard.

13 Elwin, *De Quincey*, p.120.

When engaging his reader on the 'bodily effects' of opium, De Quincey was, if not infallible, then relying on the notion of *experto crede.* When discussing 'all that has been hitherto written on the subject ... by professors of medicine, writing *ex cathedra*, De Quincey had but one emphatic criticism to give: 'Lies! lies! lies!'. He did not deny that 'some truths had been delivered to the world in regard to opium', notably on its colour, consistency, price and relative toxicity.[14] These were truths which he considered, in ironic vein, to be most weighty and commendable, but which 'exhausted the stock of knowledge as yet accumulated by man on the subject of opium'; a point reiterated by the eminent Edinburgh toxicologist Sir Robert Christison in 1826. De Quincey emphasised that he was speaking from 'the ground of a large and profound personal experience', whereas, he believed, most of 'those who have written expressly on the *materia medica*, make it evident, from the horror they express of it, that their experimental knowledge of its action is none at all'.[15] He therefore proposed that the 'worthy doctors' should allow him 'to come forward and lecture on this matter' as there seemed 'to be room for further discoveries'. And, as we shall discover, some of them did. Christison was the first to give great and grateful consideration to De Quincey's insights and experiential knowledge.[16]

In reply to an article by James Montgomery in the *Sheffield Iris* in 1821, De Quincey wrote that 'the entire confessions were designed to convey a narrative of my own experience as an opium-eater, drawn up with entire simplicity and fidelity to facts'.[17] It is only by employing hackneyed reactions to chronic opium use that twentieth-century writers on De Quincey can argue that, 'like all opium addicts [he] lied, prevaricated and romanced about his addiction'. 'Everything he says', some believe, must 'be scrutinised with a reservation' and this because he was regarded as a sick man prey to his undoubted 'infirmity'.[18] This is criticism with a twentieth-century pathological and stereotypical mien: all 'opium addicts' are the same and they are all sick. But De Quincey's language is entrenched in the Romantic idiom and must be read as such. Marilyn Butler, in *Romantics, Rebels and Reactionaries* (1981), argues that the *Confessions* are a 'clever medley of the facts of his life with fables, inconsistencies and probable lies', in that the work is subjective and intuitive. The Romantic writer differed radically from his eighteenth-century classicist predecessor by revealing a truth originating in the artist rather than attempting a mirror-like reflection of reality.[19] His work cannot survive a baldly literal, and so impoverished, reading.

The Romantic era was a period of profound change in almost all areas of human endeavour. A 'study of man' emerged from the eighteenth-century Enlightenment, the 'new science' and the cult of curiosity that investigated equally the animal kingdom,

14 De Quincey, *Confessions*, p.39.
15 Ibid., p.42.
16 See chapter 6.
17 Levine, *The Romantic Art of Confession*, p.25.
18 Hayter, *Opium and the Romantic Imagination*, p.112.
19 Butler, *Romantics, Rebels, and Reactionaries*, p.7.

plants and fossils.[20] The revolutions in political, economic, religious, scientific and social life in the late eighteenth century could not fail to influence ideas on identity and character. 'Men and women, poets and doctors, philosophers and statesmen' all clamoured to define the nature of man, and the costive eighteenth-century sensibility was transformed.[21] The 1790s brought revolutionary political works by Mary Wollstonecraft and Tom Paine; new philosophical ideas from Voltaire, d'Holbach and Condorcet crossed the channel; Malthus published *An Essay on Population* (1798), the first sociological study of major importance; men of the 'new science', such as Davy and Dalton, were dynamically experimenting with electricity, gases and combustion; Southey, Coleridge, Godwin and Blake were producing dramatic and prophetic works; and Fuseli, Turner, Gillray and Blake brought down traditional visual frontiers with representations of the demoniac and the horrors of the inner mind.[22] This was a period of intense activity and intellectual convulsion, and within this body of thought any 'dis-ease' was not always understood as exclusively physiological but also as a manifestation of the soul or personality. It was a subjective experience, related to the exploration of the self, an inversion of traditional mind–body dualism.[23]

This cultural upheaval provided the forum wherein an individual could stage a personal revolution against inherited authority and its rules. Old certitudes were undermined by social changes and scepticism became an indispensable attribute of many Romantic artists. The concept of the artist as a neurotic, socially disengaged malcontent bent on cultivating a uniquely enigmatic persona was ushered in. In the pre-Romantic eighteenth century such behaviour might have been viewed as a form of insanity, but even this became worth affecting as a form of child-like innocence combined with an almost mystical sagacity. The individual became a conduit for new ideas about human nature and ceased to be of interest merely as a conglomeration of general human characteristics.[24] Personality, as a concept, was a subject of great curiosity during the first thirty years of the nineteenth century, and this extended interest in heightened sensibility and the development of the self was manifested in a flood of biographical and confessional works. This was 'fertile ground for the cult of the isolated, introverted literary personality', and it was appropriate to this transitional 'age of opinion' and synthesis that a journal should carry in the 'new wave'. In the 1820s *The London Magazine* carried not only De Quincey's *Confessions*, but also Hazlitt's 'Table Talk' and Lamb's equally personal 'Essays of Elia'. These works represented a new kind of literary autobiography, 'more quirky than anything of the

---

20 Ibid., pp.2, 4.

21 A.K. Henderson, *Romantic Identities: Varieties of Subjectivity 1774-1830* (1996), p.166.

22 R. Holmes, *Shelley: The Pursuit* (1994), pp.8-9.

23 R. Porter, 'Medicine', in McCalman, *Oxford Companion to the Romantic Age*, pp.175-6.

24 A. Brookner, *Romanticism and its Discontents* (2000), p.iv.

kind before', and they created a bridge of understanding between the public and the 'literary genius'.[25]

De Quincey was a 'great projector of the self' and he provided the 'first memorable portrait of the modern artist, simultaneously drop-out and saint'.[26] Unmistakable honesty is discernible throughout his confessions. He was unafraid to tell it as he experienced it; he did not spare his readers either the pleasures or the pains of his addiction, nor the uplifting or degrading sensations. He saw no conflict in his contradictory experiences for they were the paradoxical results of his self-exploration.

But his work did not escape criticism, and much of that was based on moral issues rather than on a denial of his literary skill or the veracity of his experiences. He was accused of being a pernicious influence, a vile inspiration to the potential addict, and there were calls for the work to be suppressed. A letter written by Robert Southey to Samuel Cottle notes that, because of 'Mr De Quincey's book ... one who had never taken a drop of opium before, took so large a dose, for the sake of experiencing the sensations that had been described, that a very little addition to the dose might have proved fatal'.[27] When there was a fatality in 1823 a physician at the inquest reported that he had witnessed an alarming increase in such incidences 'in consequence of a little book that has been published by a man of literature, which recites many extraordinary cases of taking opium'. Four of his patients had allegedly told him that the *Confessions* had inspired their experimentation and as, he stated, 'almost every young man of practice and science had been induced to purchase this work', it was 'therefore ... of universal ill tendency'. Some, though, were persuaded against the drug by reading the book. Thomas Carlyle had read it before trying laudanum for his chronic insomnia, and he concluded that it would be 'better, a thousand times better, *die* than have anything to do with such a Devil's own drug'.[28] De Quincey was drawn into refuting all these allegations, exclaiming 'Teach opium-eating! Did I teach wine-drinking? Did I reveal the mystery of sleeping? Did I inaugurate the infirmity of laughter? ... No man is likely to adopt opium or to lay it aside in consequence of anything he may read in a book'.[29] Even so, there were still some who were at least metaphorically seduced into sampling opium half a century on, as Madison Julius Cawein's poem, 'Opium. On reading De Quincey's *Confessions of an Opium Eater*', reveals:

25 Butler, *Romantics, Rebels, and Reactionaries*, p.174.

26 Ibid., p.175.

27 Hayter, *Opium and the Romantic Imagination*, pp.105-6.

28 Lindop, *The Opium-Eater*, p.248.

29 Hayter, *Opium and the Romantic Imagination*, pp.105-6. This is an argument that Hayter believes to be 'a weak and unconvincing defence', and in doing so she again supports and echoes similar attacks, past and present, on the idea of knowledge as a corrupting and destructive agent.

> And voices, - lost in darkness, - deep that called.
> I entered. And beneath the dome's high-halled
> Immensity one forced me to my knees
> Before a blackness...[30]

De Quincey himself wrote that although the fascinating powers of the drug had often been 'admitted ... even by medical writers', these men remained 'its greatest enemies'. Their professional attempts to keep the truth to themselves, and to so monopolise and police the drug, denied people what he saw as the varied and valuable experiences to be had by its agency. As an example of medical prevarication he quoted Aswiter, an apothecary to Greenwich Hospital, who had first published his *Essay on the Effects of Opium* in 1763. The work contained an opaque attempt to explain the eminent physician Mead's evasive concern over the drug's properties:

> perhaps he thought the subject of too delicate a nature to be made common; and as many people might then indiscriminately use it, it would take from that necessary fear and caution, which should prevent their experiencing the extensive power of this drug: *for there are many properties in it, if universally known, that would habituate the use, and make it more in request with us than the Turks themselves;* the result of which knowledge must prove a general misfortune.[31]

Whenever opium was discussed 'formally or incidentally' it was De Quincey's opinion that the intoxicating effects of the drug were taken as a given, without any interpretative qualification. He himself objected to this lazy, deceptive adoption of a common idea and assured his readers that 'no quantity of opium ever did, or could intoxicate'. Laudanum might do so, he conceded, but only because of the proof spirit it contained. Opium, he insisted, resembled alcohol neither in effect nor in degree nor in kind.[32] And it was in a quantitative and particularly in a qualitative way that the two drugs differed greatly. The pleasures of wine, he thought, were to be found in the mounting sensations which tend toward a crisis and afterwards decline; those of opium, in contrast, when once generated are stationary for eight or ten hours. The former, and here he borrowed a technical distinction from medicine, 'is a case of acute pleasure', the latter of 'chronic pleasure'. But the main distinction lay in the effects on the senses and mental faculties: wine disordered them but opium, 'if taken in the proper manner', meaning in controlled moderation, could return the disciple of the 'true church' to an original state of grace, for it

> introduces amongst [the senses] the most exquisite order, legislation, and harmony. Wine robs a man of his self-possession: opium greatly invigorates it. Wine unsettles and clouds the judgement, and gives a preternatural brightness and a vivid exaltation to the contempts and the admirations, the loves and the hatreds of the drinker: opium on the

30 M.J. Cawein, 'Opium. On reading De Quincey's *Confessions of an Opium Eater*', in *The Poems*, vol. III, 'Nature Poems Tansy and Sweet Alyssum' (1908).

31 De Quincey, *Confessions*, p.4.

32 See Appendix 2 for the perceived relationship between opium and alcohol.

> contrary communicates serenity and equipoise ... and with respect to the temper and moral feelings in general, it gives simply that sort of vital warmth which is approved by the judgement, and which would probably always accompany a bodily constitution of primeval or antideluvian health. [Drinkers] swear eternal friendship, and shed tears – no mortal knows why: and the sensual creature is clearly uppermost. But the expansion of the benigner feelings incident to opium, is ... a healthy restoration to ... the impulses of a heart originally just and good.[33]

An inebriated person, in this everyman's schema, has called up that part of his or her sensual nature that is 'merely human, too often brutal' and by implication and association, shameful. But the opium-eater is not to be confused with a drunk. He rises above base carnality and 'feels that the diviner part ... is paramount; that is, the moral affections are in a state of cloudless serenity; and over all is the great light of majestic intellect'.[34] Both experiences are artificially induced or manufactured but the latter is regarded as being closest to man's nascent and therefore purest self, and is consequently superior and legitimate, covetable and easily attainable. De Quincey did not accept that this major difference was merely a matter of semantics and he dismissed the crassness of a surgeon, 'reputed a good one', who had 'taken opium largely' and who claimed to be 'drunk with opium; and *that* daily'. Though De Quincey thought it unlikely that a medical man would be unacquainted with drunkenness, he believed that a 'logical error' was being perpetrated whereby the term 'intoxication' was being used with 'too great [a] latitude'. He considered that it had been extended 'generally to all modes of nervous excitement, instead of restricting it as the expression for a specific sort ... connected with certain diagnostics'. He was searching for a specific categorisation of opium and the opium experience, a reverential recognition of the sublimity of the drug and so of his own use. He sought an elevation from the banal to the esoteric. Further, despite the classification of opium as a narcotic, he disagreed with the assumption that the elevation of the spirits produced by opium was necessarily followed by a proportionate depression. One only had to 'time the exhibition of the dose, to speak medically' so that the weight of the narcotic influence fell during a natural period of sleep.[35] He was suggesting that one could use opium to great advantage with subtle knowledge and manipulation. He initially sought acceptance that it was possible for the user to retain control of his habit, thereby being free to experience great pleasure whilst not disrupting his own or anyone else's life.

How then did De Quincey himself come to be addicted? Why did he never find himself free of it, and why did he come to lament it? He admitted that he was often asked these questions and wished to refute the allegation, commonly put to him, that he must have brought upon himself all the sufferings that he recorded, 'by a long course of indulgence ... purely for the sake of creating an artificial state of pleasurable excitement'. It was true, he wrote, that for nearly ten years he did

33 De Quincey, *Confessions*, p.41.

34 Ibid.

35 Ibid., p.6.

'occasionally take opium for the ... exquisite pleasure' it gave him but, in the first instance, he strenuously maintained that he had taken it for a respectable medicinal purpose, to mitigate pain 'in the severest degree'.[36]

In London during the autumn of 1804, at the age of eighteen and after a picaresque adolescence, he took his first dose of opium and he continued to take it until his death at the age of seventy-four.[37] For three weeks he had been in agony, suffering from excruciating rheumatic pains of the head and face, until he bumped into an acquaintance, a man, 'if man he was', who recommended opium. De Quincey felt that the druggist who subsequently dispensed the tincture to him was nothing less than an 'unconscious minister of celestial pleasures'. He seemed mortal enough, and 'dull and stupid', but had evidently been 'sent down to earth on a special mission' to the distressed young man. For, on returning home, and within an hour of taking the prescribed quantity, he experienced 'an Apocalypse of the world within'. That his terrible pain had vanished was 'a trifle ... this negative effect was swallowed up in the immensity of those positive effects' which opened up before him, 'in the abyss of divine enjoyment thus revealed'. His first dose had miraculously revealed to him 'the secret of happiness', a secret, moreover, which could 'be bought for a penny, and carried in the waistcoat pocket: portable ecstasies ... corked up in a pint bottle'. But, despite his youthful, delirious eulogies, De Quincey, with experience and hindsight, gave his readers the grim warning that 'nobody will laugh long who deals much with opium'.[38]

Throughout the *Confessions* we discern the dichotomous nature of the opium response. During the ten years following his dramatic introduction to the drug De Quincey took it sporadically, perhaps only once every three weeks on an 'opium evening'. These 'debauches' were fixed beforehand, usually for a Tuesday or a Saturday night, either at the Opera house amongst the wealthy and civilised or wandering through 'all the markets and other parts of London to which the poor resort ... for laying out their wages'. It was only much later that De Quincey would 'venture to call every day ... for "*a glass of laudanum negus, warm, and without sugar*"'.[39] In the meantime, however, he believed himself to be suffering from, among other things, a nascent form of tuberculosis, and he took opium sometimes medicinally and sometimes in a self-proclaimed 'dillettante' [sic] fashion. By 1812 he was living as a "*gentleman*' and indulged his predilection on Saturday nights, claiming he had never felt better in his life than in the spring of that year. This he ascribed to the 'excellent suggestion' of his physician, a Dr Buchan, that he should be 'particularly careful not to take above five-and-twenty ounces of laudanum'. Depending on the quality of opium this amount could have constituted up to, if not slightly more than, the three grams of morphine that would today be considered

36 Ibid.

37 Elwin, *De Quincey*, p.10.

38 De Quincey, *Confessions*, p.39.

39 Ibid., p.44. Negus is a drink of port or sherry with hot water, sweetened and spiced, and was first concocted by a Colonel Negus in the early eighteenth century.

a substantial amount to tolerate.[40] De Quincey referred to this as 'moderation and temperate use of the article', following the traditional humoral philosophy on health and well-being. And, with 'intervals between every indulgence', he found that it was not necessary 'to make opium ... an article of daily diet'. At this point he still considered himself 'ignorant and unsuspicious of the avenging terrors which opium has in store for those who abuse its lenity'.[41]

But illness overtook him again in 1813 and he fell prey to a 'most appalling irritation of the stomach', the point in his narrative on which the gist of his confessions hinged. He entered into a struggle between his constant suffering and chronic opium use on the one hand, and on the other the additional pain he would feel on being shamefully accused of weakness and self-indulgence. He asked his readers to believe only that he could resist no longer, for 'at the time [he] began to take opium daily, [he] could not have done otherwise'. 'I cannot face misery', he wrote, 'whether my own or not ... and am little capable of encountering present pain for the sake of any reversionary benefit'.[42] From the onset of his illness De Quincey considered himself to be 'a regular and confirmed opium-eater, of whom to ask whether on any particular day he had or had not taken opium, would be to ask whether his lungs had performed respiration, or the heart fulfilled its functions'. He wanted it to be fully understood exactly what he was, to brave any shame he felt or any heaped upon him. No one would be able to persuade him to give up his 'little golden receptacle of the pernicious drug'. No 'moralists or surgeons ... whatever be their pretensions or skill in their respective lines of practice' could now hope that he would be persuaded to countenance an 'abstinence from opium'.[43]

There was no attempt to mask the experience or to make it more acceptable, palatable or reasonable to the uninitiated and uninformed. He wrote as though thinking aloud, rather than in consideration of who might be, as it were, listening. And he believed that had he stopped to imagine what might be deemed 'proper' he would have begun to doubt the wisdom of telling his story at all.[44] That much of his account appears to be incomprehensibly bizarre only adds to its veracity. De Quincey remarks, for example, that only a little while before his plunge into constant use he had, 'strange as it may sound', reduced his dose 'suddenly, and without any considerable effort, from 320 grains of opium (*i.e.* eight thousand drops of laudanum) per day, to forty grains'. He spent the ensuing, 'intercalary' year taking opium every evening, writing, reading and once more experiencing the 'feelings of pleasure [that] expanded themselves to all around [him]'. He had reached that plateau of use that sustained many other opium-takers throughout long and productive lives, some of which will be touched on later. This period, when he knew 'happiness, both in a solid and a liquid shape, both boiled and unboiled, both East India and Turkey', did

40 See Appendix 1.

41 De Quincey, *Confessions*, pp.51-2.

42 Ibid., p.53.

43 Ibid., p.54.

44 Ibid., p.61.

not last, however, and he succumbed to the 'Illiad of woes' which were the terrible 'pains of opium'.[45]

The 'Circean spells of opium' that infatuated and 'degraded' De Quincey between 1813 and 1817 left him in a dormant state in which he felt he existed only by virtue of his suffering. The dreams, waking and sleeping, that he experienced were the most immediate cause of his 'acutest suffering'. 'Incubus and night-mare' drove him into 'an oppression as of madness' accompanied by spiritual, moral and physical terrors. Temporal and spatial distortions, 'deep-seated anxiety and gloomy melancholy, such as [were] wholly incommunicable by words' tormented his days and nights.[46] His consequent self-neglect, incapacity and feebleness reduced his practical and dutiful life but, perhaps tragically, not his 'moral sensibilities or aspirations'. 'Powerless as an infant', unable even to attempt to rise from his couch, he himself, at this juncture, likened his condition to a sickness. But this was a metaphor for his descriptive and debilitating state: it was merely a simulacrum of disease.[47] He suffered, but he did not consider himself to be truly pathologically ill.

The original edition of the *Confessions* conveyed De Quincey's object in writing as a wish to 'display the marvellous agency of opium, whether for pleasure or for pain', the opium and not the opium-eater being 'the true hero of the tale'. But he felt bound to satisfy the curiosity of others as to his continuing relationship with the drug. The pains by this time had come far to outweigh the pleasures and it was the tortures that attended his attempts to abstain that caused him to keep taking his heroic amount of opium. It was 'a choice only of evils': he realised he would die if he continued and so determined to die by leaving it off, 'if that should be required'. And so he commenced gradually to reduce his daily dose, even though after four months he was 'still agitated, writhing, throbbing, palpitating, shattered', deriving no effective relief from any other medicines. Some thirty years later the 1856 edition of his *Confessions* recounts his 'four several times' renunciation and resumption of the habit and his lack of excuse for his failures. He would acknowledge only that, of the two evil states he had experienced, the taking of opium was 'very much the least' and that he resumed his consumption through 'enlightened and deliberate judgment'.[48] He thereafter maintained a small daily habit and the physician who attended his last illness in 1859 believed that it had at least sustained his mind in defiance of his poor physical condition when 'life was a mere misery ... from nerves', rendered endurable only by opium.[49]

The cause of his death is unknown but was ascribed 'rather to exhaustion of the system than to specific disease' and the post-mortem examination revealed that his 'organs [had] received no damage from his prolonged opium eating indeed

45 Ibid., pp.58, 61.
46 Ibid., p.66.
47 Ibid., p.67.
48 Ibid., p.11.
49 Elwin, *De Quincey*, pp.133, 138.

being exceptionally sound'.[50] Nevertheless opium-eaters reading the work had been encouraged to take consolation from De Quincey's efforts to rid himself of his bondage. Opium could be renounced, he had written, and 'without greater sufferings than an ordinary resolution may support'. The trick was to reduce the dose gently and avoid aggravating the inevitable physical and mental pains.[51] The original purpose of the tale, that other opium-eaters might be taught to 'fear and tremble', had been supplanted by a greater empiricism and a resigned understanding of his condition.

De Quincey believed he was rendering a service to a great many others who perhaps suffered as he did. But who were they, this 'whole class of opium-eaters'? He listed some he knew of, either directly or indirectly, within his own 'small class of English society'. Some were distinguished by their talents, some by their eminent position, some by their eloquence and benevolence. He named Samuel Taylor Coleridge as well as William Wilberforce, Dr Isaac Milner (Dean of Carlisle), Lord Chancellor Erskine, and, including some anonymous 'philosophers and politicians', he suggested that there were 'many others, hardly less known, whom it would be tedious to mention'.[52]

Opium, in dry pill form, was prescribed for William Wilberforce by his physician, a Dr Warren, to alleviate 'debility, loss of appetite, feverishness, and recurrent diarrhoea'. This amalgamation of symptoms, probably exacerbated by his demanding political life, was treated with the most reliable panacea in the late eighteenth-century pharmacopoeia. When, after a few years of regular use, he wished to stop taking the drug, Dr Isaac Milner, who had also relied 'heavily on opium' for many years, sent him an unequivocal letter telling him to 'be not afraid of the *habit* of such medicine, the *habit* of growling guts is infinitely worse'. Milner argued that there was 'nothing injurious to the constitution in the medicines and if you use them all your life there is no great harm. But paroxysms of laxity or pain leave permanent evil'.[53]

Wilberforce was taking five grains daily by 1796 and by 1818, thirty years after his first prescription, his diary reveals that the dose was 'still as it has long been' and not 'commonly exceeded' a pill three times a day, each of four grains. This is not a substantial amount, equivalent to perhaps 76 milligrams of morphine a day, but sufficient to have him 'forced to lie in bed, great sneezing and other signs of spasm with sweating' if he missed his night-time dose. Wilberforce himself recommended laudanum and opium, and Dr Perceval the proprietary opiate 'Black Drop', to Lord Harrowby, Foreign Secretary in 1804, who suffered intolerable and constant headaches following a fall.[54] These highly respectable gentlemen of virtue and nobility saw no shame in their addiction, nor in their recommending regular opium-taking to others, rather they regarded it as an obvious and necessary evil, if paradoxically, a beneficent one.

---

50 Lindop, *The Opium-Eater*, p.387.

51 Elwin, *De Quincey*, p.227.

52 Ibid., pp.16-17.

53 J. Pollock, *William Wilberforce* (1977), pp.78-84.

54 Ibid.

De Quincey thought opium-eaters to be 'a very numerous class indeed', having extrapolated out from those he was aware of, for 'if one class, comparatively so limited, could furnish so many scores of cases, it was a natural inference that the entire population of England would furnish a proportionable number'. Any doubts about this he erased from his own mind when he heard evidence, from the geographically dispersed London druggists he frequented, as to their extensive clientele. The druggists also, it is valuable to note, told him they had to go to a great deal of trouble in their attempts to distinguish potential suicides from those customers 'to whom habit had rendered opium necessary'.[55] They would refuse the drug to the suicidal whose actions would also, of course, invite the scrutiny of the coroner's courts, but they appeared, in a professional sense, to recognise and accept the need of, or to feel perhaps more merciful towards, the *habitué*. Were the former deranged sinners who might bring opprobrium upon themselves and others, but the latter seen as proto-medical cases whose disease of habit would have to be endured, its worst symptoms mollified with narcotic gratification? Or perhaps the *habitué* was simply, and obviously, a more desirable and profitable customer.

Samuel Taylor Coleridge and the experience of addiction

Whilst De Quincey lived for years under opium's spell without the ministrations of any physician, Coleridge was one such medical case. At least he thought of himself as one and was similarly regarded and treated as a patient by his doctors. De Quincey-ite experiences of opium-derived cerebral and sensual pleasures were denied by Coleridge who, though he referred to his first doses as delivering him into 'divine' repose, spent much of his life cursing the 'Poison' and his own wretched need of it.[56] His wife, Sarah, cursed it too, lamenting that she 'should be a very, very happy Woman if it were not for a few things – and my husband's ill health stands at the head of these evils!'[57] Coleridge's later notebooks say very little on the pleasures of opium but he wrote a great deal on the physical and psychological pains of leaving off the drug.[58]

Both men, by their own accounts, had begun taking opium when afflicted with illness and pain, both mental and physical. In a letter dated December 1796 Coleridge noted that he had been forced to make 'frequent use of Laudanum' to alleviate a rheumatic complaint and a 'depression of the animal Spirits'. He was also 'obliged to take Laudanum almost every night' during March 1796 when he was 'tottering

55 Elwin, *De Quincey*, pp.16-17.

56 H.J. Jackson, ed., *Samuel Taylor Coleridge: Selected Letters* (1987), pp.38, 175.

57 K. Jones, *A Passionate Sisterhood: The Sisters, Wives, and Daughters of the Lake Poets* (1997), p.150.

58 R. Holmes, *Coleridge: Darker Reflections* (1998), p.12. Holmes argues that Coleridge's addiction might be considered an 'emotional state' reflecting an imaginative dependency on close human relationships; that 'Love and Opium are sometimes interchangeable substances in Coleridge's mind and body'.

on the edge of madness – [his] mind overbalanced on the contra side of Happiness'. His wife was dangerously ill with a threatened miscarriage and there were blunders and frustrations in his public life that he had to deal with at the same time. Opium provided undoubted comfort and relief to his emotional distress and difficulties.[59] In his letters to friends and confidantes during 1796 Coleridge wrote of 'intolerable pain from my right temple to the tip of my right shoulder … I was nearly frantic, and ran about the house naked, endeavouring by every means to excite sensations in different parts of my body, and so to weaken the enemy'. His medical attendant decided his condition was 'altogether nervous, and that it originates either in severe application, or excessive anxiety'. The patient thought that 'in excessive anxiety, I believe it might originate … I take twenty-five drops of laudanum every five hours, the ease and *spirits* gained by which have enabled me to write [to] you'. On the back of this letter the recipient, his publisher Joseph Cottle, had written despairingly and perhaps in exasperation, 'Oh! That S.T.C. had never taken more than 25 drops each dose'.[60]

Writing to his brother two years later about an indisposition that originated in a toothache and thence 'affected my eye, my eye my stomach, my stomach my head; and the consequence was a general fever', Coleridge found that laudanum alone provided 'a spot of inchantment, a green spot of fountains, & flowers & trees, in the very heart of a waste of Sands!'[61] In the midst of his later desperate struggles with the drug he wrote that he had been 'seduced into the ACCURSED Habit ignorantly', that, when suffering with swollen knee-joints, he had read in a medical journal of a similar case cured by the internal and external use of laudanum. On experimenting he found that it acted on him 'like a charm, like a miracle!', but as the 'unusual stimulus subsided – the complaint returned'. The 'supposed remedy' was resorted to again and it set in motion a 'dreary history', a continuing cycle of need and gratification. His desire for opium, he protested repeatedly, was produced by '*Terror & Cowardice* of PAIN & sudden Death, not (so help me God!) by any temptation of pleasure, or expectation or desire of exciting pleasurable sensations'.[62]

Pleasure or no, Coleridge's account of the influence of opium-induced dreams on his writing of 'Kubla Khan' (1797) revealed what was to him a non-shameful dimension to opium use: the drug's role in the act of imaginative creation. His ideas of visionary composition through opium-induced reveries found greater popular expression with the publication of De Quincey's *Suspira De Profundis* (1849) and were much imitated by others, Baudelaire and Cocteau for example. Others, such as Charles Lamb, took satirical advantage of his ideas. Lamb, in his essay 'Witches and other Night Fears' (1821), included this piece of burlesque:

> The poverty of my dreams mortifies me. There is Coleridge, at his will can conjure up icy domes, and pleasure-houses for Kubla Kahn, and Abyssinian maids, and songs of Abora,

59 L. Hanson, *The Life of S.T. Coleridge: The Early Years* (1938), p.101.
60 Ibid., pp.132, 452.
61 Jackson, *Samuel Taylor Coleridge*, pp.38, 67.
62 Ibid., pp.173-9, 269.

> and caverns … to solace his night's solitudes – when I cannot muster a fiddle … An old gentleman, a friend of mine, and a humourist, used to carry this notion so far, that when he saw any stripling of his acquaintance with ambitions of becoming a poet, his first question would be: 'Young man, what sort have dreams have you?'[63]

But Coleridge felt that, through the drug, the imagination or 'shaping power' still operated in the writer's mind, so that the resulting work could never be merely 'phantasmagoria'.[64] De Quincey was in agreement when he wrote that the man who talks of oxen would dream of oxen and nothing more.[65] The idea that opium might inspire great works has provoked some hostility amongst twentieth-century commentators. Molly Lefebure's *Samuel Taylor Coleridge: A Bondage of Opium* (1974) flatly denies Coleridge's own accounts and insists that the drug destroyed his life and talents.[66] But the poet had a far more perceptive eye on opium than this and understood its action as an agent of the imagination, anticipating the twentieth-century medical view that the effects of a drug will depend as much on the psychological make-up and the environment of the user as upon the properties of the substance. It is now assumed to be a fallacy that there are predictable or measurable effects that manifest themselves in all users.[67]

Many physicians attended to the effects of Coleridge's habit which by 1814 had become excessive and reached up to six grams of opium a day: 'in twenty-four hours, a whole quart of laudanum!', according to Cottle, 'besides great quantities of liquor'.[68] But his habit was not referred to as an addiction. Dorothy Wordsworth, for example, said he had a 'practice', whilst Sara Hutchinson called it a 'passion' for opium.[69] Nevertheless he was consequently beset by physical weakness, aches, feverishness, and constipation from taking the drug, as well as diarrhoea from leaving it off. He sent for a brass 'Clyster Machine' from Everall and Wilson's of St James's Street so that he could administer his own enemas and he experimented with various 'recipes', including a dilute laudanum mixture of five pounds of quince juice to a pound of opium with cinnamon, nutmeg, cloves and saffron. His condition rendered him often 'thoroughly *be-belzebubbed*'.[70] In a letter to his friend Morgan, in May 1814, Coleridge wrote of the efforts made by Doctors Tuthill and Daniel to control all his self-dosing and of their suggestion that he might 'be removed to a place of confinement, or at all events have a Keeper'. He himself wished fervently

63 Charles Lamb, 'Witches and other Night Fears' (1821), in E. Dowden, ed., *The Correspondence of Robert Southey with Caroline Bowles. To which are added: Correspondence with Shelley, and Southey's Dreams* (1881), p.x, n.1.

64 Holmes, *Coleridge*, pp.434-5.

65 De Quincey, *Confessions*, p.5.

66 M. Lefebure, *Samuel Taylor Coleridge: A Bondage of Opium* (1974), p.32

67 M. Glossop, 'The Effects of Drugs' in Coomber, *Drugs and Drug Use*, pp. 24-5.

68 Holmes, *Coleridge*, p.355.

69 J. Ford, *Coleridge on Dreaming: Romanticism and the Medical Imagination* (1998), p.207, n.2.

70 Ibid., pp.103-4, 357, 365.

for a place, perhaps in a private madhouse, where he 'could procure nothing but what a Physician thought proper, & where a medical attendant could be constantly with [him] for two or three months (in less than that time Life or Death would be determined) then there might be Hope'.[71] Such an arrangement would remove all personal responsibility for his condition, break his habit and perhaps also diminish his sense of failure and weakness. In 1816 Morgan introduced him to a new physician, Joseph Adams, who had some knowledge of chronic opium use. Adams wrote to James Gillman, a member of the Royal College of Surgeons, the man to whom Coleridge was to abdicate responsibility for his drug use and who cared for the poet until his death in July 1834:

> Dear Sir, a very learned, but in one respect an unfortunate gentleman, has applied to me on a singular occasion. He has for several years been in the habit of taking large quantities of opium. For some time past, he has been in vain endeavouring to break himself off. It is apprehended his friends are not firm enough, lest he should suffer by suddenly leaving it off, though he is conscious of the contrary; and has proposed to me to submit himself to any regime, however severe. With this view, he wishes to fix himself in the house of some medical gentleman, who will have courage to refuse him any laudanum, and under whose assistance, should he be the worse for it, he may be relieved ... I could think of no one so readily as yourself.[72]

Gillman was a young married man with two small children, and was understandably initially very wary of accepting into his house a man with such an entrenched habit, no matter how learned or respectable he might be. Moreover he had spoken with Adams of the possible 'frightful consequences' of a detoxification regime, having heard of 'the failure of Mr Wilberforce's case, under an eminent physician at Bath, in addition to which, the doctor [Adams] gave me an account of several others within his own knowledge'.[73] But he found Coleridge to be genial, charming, courteous and quite unexpectedly candid and self-analytical about his habit and behaviour. Gillman was given to understand that 'unless watched carefully' Coleridge could not promise that, 'with regard to this detested Poison', he would not 'be capable of *acting* a Lie' nor that '*Evasion*, and the cunning of a specific madness' would not rule him completely.[74]

Arrangements were made and Coleridge moved into the surgeon's house where, in the facetiously dismissive words of Lamb, he was 'under the medical care of a Mr Gillman (*Killman?*) a Highgate Apothecary, where he *plays at leaving off Laudanum*'. From this point on there was no attempt to conceal the habit: had he not anyway begun it '*unwittingly*' in the course of illness? His physician knew the condition to be 'far from unique' and remarked that few had 'dared blacken Mr Wilberforce's good name on this account' despite his having 'been for years under

71 Jackson, *Samuel Taylor Coleridge*, p.175.

72 Holmes, *Coleridge*, p.424.

73 Ibid., pp.427-8.

74 Jackson, *Samuel Taylor Coleridge*, p.181.

the same necessity'. One might, in his experience, 'talk with any eminent druggist or medical practitioner, especially at the West End of the town, concerning the frequency of this calamity among men and women of eminence'.[75]

Coleridge's social life and opium-taking was significantly curtailed by his 'incarceration' which, on at least one occasion, he sought to alleviate with a foiled attempt at smuggling in laudanum with some literary proofs. His withdrawal from the drug led him into sensations of 'indefinite *Fear*' or nervous anxiety that he fought against, taking only his few prescribed drops, though 'more', he wrote irritably, 'would have been better'. This prescription exacerbated his extreme nervous restlessness but, nonetheless, allowed him to 'break the commencing Cycle before the actual Craving came on'.[76] Although he never entirely succeeded in leaving off his opium Coleridge was 'transformed' by the regulation and discipline of Gillman's regime. His 'literary career had an extraordinary second-birth' despite the fears of some of his friends who had suspected that without opium Coleridge would lose his inspiration. They accused the attending physicians of attempting to rob him of his muse and his talent. Southey went as far as to suggest cynically that Gillman was callously and calculatingly 'speculating' on the poet, 'hoping to ride his reputation with notoriety and practice', having deliberately isolated him from his friends and by getting him 'largely in debt to him' through actually maintaining his 'habits of opium'.[77]

Coleridge continued to describe his condition as an almost unbearable misery, a physiological collapse and a psychological ruin that could only be remedied by more opium. There was always that moment, that 'direful moment', when his pulse began to fluctuate, his heart to palpitate and an 'intolerable Restlessness & incipient Bewilderment' would come over him. To Cottle, who had written in 1814 exhorting him to abandon opium, Coleridge replied that no one could expect him to rouse himself any more than could a man paralysed in both arms be successfully advised to rub them briskly and so be cured: 'Alas! (he would reply) that I cannot move my arms is my Complaint & my misery'. He believed his 'Case [was] a species of madness … a derangement, an utter impotence of the *Volition*'.[78] All 'intellectual Faculties' and 'moral feelings, reason, understanding, and senses' were 'perfectly sane and vigorous' but still, he felt, he 'may yet have been mad', for:

> [by] the long long Habit of the accursed Poison my Volition (by which I mean the faculty *instrumental* to the Will, and by which alone the Will can realize itself – its Hands, Legs, & Feet, as it were) was compleatly deranged, at times frenzied, dissevered itself from the Will, & became an independent faculty: so that I was perpetually in the state, in which you may have seen paralytic Persons, who attempting to push a step forward in one direction are violently forced round to the opposite. I was sure that no ease, much less pleasure, would ensue: nay I was certain of an accumulation of pain. But tho' there was no prospect,

75 Holmes, *Coleridge*, pp.444-5.
76 Ibid., pp.429-30.
77 Ibid., pp.432-3.
78 Jackson, *Samuel Taylor Coleridge*, pp.173-9.

> no gleam of Light before, an indefinite indescribable Terror as with a scourge of ever restless, ever coiling and coiling Serpents, drove me from behind.[79]

If he was not to consider himself mad perhaps he might argue that he was not fully responsible for 'certain dream devils or damned Souls that play pranks with me … by the operation of a cathartic Pill or from the want of one'. For he was, he wrote in a letter to James Gillman in 1824, 'half-tempted' to regard their whisperings and conversations as external and only 'half-appropriated' by his 'Soul' and 'Sensorium'.[80] He understood that his will, his self, remained untouched but the mechanics of it, his volition, was corrupted. This self-diagnosis was not expressly a pathological nor a psychological one and it was only towards the end of the nineteenth century that such a distinction would be attempted.

Coleridge's correspondence constituted his body of confessional work wherein he castigated himself and revealed his dread mortification. Acknowledged and agonised over, he understood his lies and deceptions as human fallibility, an inescapable curse cast by the opium that tainted his true nature. His recent biographer, Richard Holmes, divines powerful religious and philosophical elements in Coleridge's confessions which have their roots in his belief in a fundamental corruption of human will: a derivation of original sin that allowed him both to acknowledge and to accept his own guilt.[81] This rhetoric of fallenness was pervasive throughout the nineteenth century, generating tensions between materialist and idealist understandings of the self and of moral action, between social identities and aesthetic ideals. Materialists adhered to a doctrine of necessity that rendered human action mechanical and governable by laws of causation. A materialist understanding of the self was embedded in medical doctrine and in the other influential sciences of psychology, phrenology and physiognomy.[82] Idealists, such as Coleridge and those who followed German romanticism and idealism, subscribed to the notion of character as self-created and not beholden to a scientific, mechanised or 'industrialised' interpretation.[83]

Coleridge appeared almost to revel in the guilt and shame he felt at the squandering of his talents and his feelings of 'utter nothingness, impotence, & worthlessness'. He would willingly, he wrote, have been 'trodden & spit upon, if by any means it might be an atonement for the direful guilt'.[84] His letters on opium read like a litany of desperation and shame, analytical and excoriating. They do not deserve the glib criticism of such as Lefebure or Hayter who have refused to 'believe what he tells us about it' and who will not give credit or trust to either his memory or his truthfulness.

79 Ibid., letter to J. J. Morgan, 14 May 1814, p.175.

80 Ford, *Coleridge on Dreaming*, p.149.

81 Holmes, *Coleridge*, p.356.

82 See chapter 7.

83 A. Anderson, *Tainted Souls and Painted Faces: The Rhetoric of Fallenness in Victorian Culture* (1993), pp.1, 3, 34.

84 Letters to Cottle and Morgan, 1814, Jackson, *Samuel Taylor Coleridge*, pp.179, 181.

They 'know', with anachronistic twentieth-century certainty that all 'addicts' lie.[85] What Coleridge knew, and freely admitted to himself and to others, were the existence of the lies which supported his craving, that 'for years' the 'anguish of [his] spirit [had] been indescribable' and the 'conscience of [his] GUILT far far worse than all!' And the worst was, he wrote, that:

> in *exact proportion* to the *importance* and *urgency* of any Duty was it, as of a fatal necessity, sure to be neglected: because it added to the Terror ... In exact proportion, as I *loved* any person or persons more than others, & would have sacrificed my Life for them, were *they* sure to be the most barbarously mistreated by silence, absence, or breach of promise ... I have in this one dirty business of Laudanum an hundred times deceived, tricked, nay actively & consciously LIED. – And yet *all* these vices are so opposite to my nature, that but for this *free-agency-annihilating* Poison. I verily believe that I should have suffered myself to have been cut to pieces rather than have committed any of them.[86]

Coleridge's deeply felt and articulate diatribes against his habit fit perfectly well with his occasional and apparently flippant remarks and off-handedness; the drug delivered both its pleasures and its pains; it drove its users into ambivalent behaviour and paradoxical thought. It is too clumsy, too prosaic, to make the assumption that an addict cannot be believed because he or she records such varied attitudes; the reality was and is far more complex. For 'more than 30 years' Coleridge's acknowledged 'self-poisoning' and his 'craving for the Poison' had 'been the guilt, debasement, and misery of [his] Existence'.[87] Could he have written a more emphatic denunciation of himself and his need? No, but neither did he hesitate to be cheered when the wife of the landscape painter William Collins responded to his misery with 'Mr Coleridge, do not cry; if the opium really does you any good, and you *must* have it, why do you not go and get it?' He was later heard to exclaim how very sensible this woman was.[88]

Coleridge's sometimes arrogant ambivalence towards his opium addiction was apparent in his approach towards medicine in general. He remarked in a note to a paper by Thomas Beddoes in 1813 that, 'no Disease was ever yet cured, but merely suspended', and seventeen years later, in response to a letter from Southey, he wrote that 'all remedies without exception are in their effects Diseases'.[89] Coleridge was a 'cultivated non-professional student of medicine', with a good understanding of the medical systems of his time which he interpreted as being intimately connected with metaphysical questions.[90]

Coleridge's and De Quincey's experiences of, and writings on, the effects of opium elucidate intoxication in precise detail, 'a notoriously difficult thing to do'.

---

85 Hayter, *Opium and the Romantic Imagination*, p.195.

86 Ibid.

87 Jackson, *Samuel Taylor Coleridge*, pp.173-9, 269.

88 Hayter, *Opium and the Romantic Imagination*, pp.255-8.

89 H. De Almeida, *Romantic Medicine and John Keats* (1991), pp.138, 141.

90 N. Vickers, *Coleridge and the Doctors 1795-1806* (2004), p.1.

Grappling with the inherent subjectivity of the material presents enormous problems of veracity for, just as 'no two drug experiences are entirely alike ... nor, of course, are any two drug-takers'.[91] But the very communication of the uniqueness of their addiction experiences rested in a universal language, which was recognised throughout the nineteenth century and beyond. Their works were seminal and formed a basis of understanding for the layperson and for the medical profession; they influenced the overall social and scientific attitudes towards the chronic use of opium. So, what then of the experiences of those that followed them and their path, those that the medical profession eventually came to see as 'diseased'? How did they come to illuminate theories of addiction, how did they differ from or obscure them, and in what ways did they support or conform to them? What routes into long-term opium use were there and what responses did this behaviour elicit, both from the user and from those close to him or her? And how, finally, was all this interpreted and presented by those who indulged in it or were otherwise affected by it?

91 W. Self, 'Introduction' to M. Ageyev, *Novel With Cocaine* (1999), p.xi.

Chapter Three

Interpretations of Nineteenth-Century Addiction: Fact and Fiction

> Experience is never limited, and it is never complete; it is an immense sensibility.
>
> Henry James, *The Art of Fiction Partial Portraits*

The double-edged sword of opium

Reactions to opium addiction, by the *habitués* themselves and by observers, took many and various forms. But whether the ubiquitous use of the drug produced popular derision, fear, pity or disgust, it was the intensely personal experience of opium that was at the root of any representation or interpretation of its use. That there were pleasures to be enjoyed was undeniable, but there was also a terrible truth in the despair and loss that was experienced by addicts and by the families and friends who struggled with the effects of the habit alongside them. These experiences and trials of addiction were given graphic presentation via the culturally influential medium of respectable Victorian fiction, informing and inspiring character and plot in political and moral fashion. The aim of this chapter is to show how images of addiction were presented and employed by popular authors, and how these portrayals had their provenance in a familiar reality.

Much of Victorian popular fiction, particularly from the mid-century onwards, had a sharply topical content, and where melodramatic inflation was employed it was presented with reflective realism. Authors such as George Eliot and Charles Dickens presented a vision of society, holding up a mirror-image of private and public life and revealing an underlying concept of culture as an 'organic legacy', frequently imbued with deep moral intention.[1] The 1840s and 50s had produced a mass of information on social issues, and the reading public was fully aware of the context in which the main body of social-problem fiction was written. The more that was known and understood about society and human behaviour, the easier it was to see it as an interconnecting whole: the model society promoted by the cultural

1 P. Coveney, 'Introduction' to George Eliot, *Felix Holt, The Radical* (1866), p.11; D. Craig, 'Introduction' to Charles Dickens, *Hard Times* (1854), p.12.

evolutionist Herbert Spencer; and the 'social and moral web' used as a structural device by writers such as Eliot, Dickens and Wilkie Collins.[2]

Professor Asa Briggs, discussing Eliot's *Middlemarch* (1871-72), argued that, in many ways the Victorian novel is an historical document. It is a record of the times which can be used as a primary source in that many social and political aspects of the popular novel persisted into, or had their analogues in, wider Victorian society.[3] Accounts of addiction, as an appeal to the imagination and as used overwhelmingly as a device to convey misery, loss, and degradation, are liberally scattered throughout the literature of the nineteenth century and were frequently based on the firsthand experiences of the writers. The reading public was becoming increasingly familiar with opiate addiction and with the obloquy or pity that accompanied it.

Late eighteenth- and early nineteenth-century literary experiences of addiction

Edmund Oliver, Charles Lloyd's picaresque novel published in 1798, is widely regarded as a *roman à clef,* addressing the drug habit and character of Coleridge, whom Lloyd had initially admired but later came to despise. Lloyd was himself an opium addict and was to take refuge with De Quincey in the Lake District while dosing himself for 'irritability and spasmodic affections of incipient insanity'.[4] He described Edmund Oliver as 'a character of excessive sensibility, and impetuous desires' who could only quiet the 'gnawing of [his] heart' by taking opium to 'stupefy and corporealize' his fervid emotions. In volume one of the novel, Lloyd, acknowledging the powers of opium, had Oliver give a confessional account of how he fell into the 'snares laid for [his] intoxication' and sank deep into the 'delirium of the sensual gratification'. The hero continued his litany of sorrow describing feelings familiar to all opium users:

> Yet at this time I felt that every virtue, even though it cost me the severest self-denial, was possible for me could I find one being to sympathize with me in the performance of it … often after the phrensies of intoxication, or the mad pleasures of an illicit commerce, in the hours of succeeding vacancy, and the freedom from the slavery of appetite, have I cursed myself in agony of spirit! … I have melted down hours in an indescribable trance … and I started up groaning and gnashing my teeth![5]

In the eighteenth century, at different times throughout his life, Samuel Johnson had suffered agonies of spirit through using opium to relieve sickness and sorrow. His frequent self-reflections had 'wrought in him a persuasion, that the evils of human life preponderated against the enjoyments of it', and this opinion he would

---

2 K. Flint, *The Victorian Novelist: Social Problems and Social Change* (1987), pp.1-2.

3 Cited in W.J. Harvey, 'Introduction' to Eliot, *Middlemarch* (1871-72), pp.17-18.

4 Hayter, *Opium and the Romantic Imagination*, p.27.

5 Charles Lloyd, *Edmund Oliver* (1798), 1, pp.x, 17, 18, 247.

frequently enforce by an observation on 'the general use of narcotics in all parts of the world'.[6] Johnson had what his biographer, Sir John Hawkins, called a strong propensity to the use of opium, which apparently increased as he advanced in years. He was first induced to use it for 'relief against watchfulness', but when it became habitual it was the 'means of a positive pleasure, and as such was resorted to by him whenever any depression of spirits made it necessary'. He usually took his opium on a spoon against the side of a cup half full of some liquid with which he washed the bitter substance down. 'With so few resources of delight', Hawkins believed, it was not to be wondered at if, after being widowed and suffering a deep, prolonged melancholy, Johnson indulged his habit freely.[7] Illness and melancholy, *pace* De Quincey, were the ubiquitous bedfellows of addiction, revealing themselves as both cause and symptom.

A desire to escape the vicissitudes of life led many to a narcotic relief where they enjoyed a blissful but temporary asylum. Consider Percy Bysshe Shelley's thoughts on his own opium habit, written in a letter to his friend William Godwin in the winter of 1817-18:

> My feelings at intervals are of a deadly and torpid kind, or awakened to a state of such unnatural & keen excitement that only to instance the organ of sight, I find the very blades of grass & the boughs of distant trees present themselves to me with microscopical distinctness. Towards evening I sink into a state of lethargy & inanimation, & often remain for hours on the sofa between sleep & waking a prey to the most painful irritability of thought. Such with little intermission is my condition.[8]

During the previous three years Shelley had felt 'obliged … to take a quantity of laudanum', hoping to alleviate his suffering from fierce nervous tension and terrible headaches. He had done this 'very unwillingly and reluctantly' and it was a presentiment of what was to come. Soon troubled by 'deep depression and self-doubt' and disturbed by the manifestation of 'strange, deliberately devilish ways [and] a furious temper', Shelley's opium habit, like De Quincey's and Coleridge's, began to permeate both his life and his work. That he was plagued by what were regarded as excessive sensibilities and an abnormal excitation of his nerves, diagnosed as 'severe erethism', was taken as read by his contemporaries; that his condition should be both relieved and exacerbated by the workings of an opium habit seemed just as unsurprising.[9] Hopelessness was a recurring emotional reaction where chronic opium use had invited misery into the lives of addicts and their loved ones. There could be no escaping the deathly connection between the 'dream-creating', physiologically and psychologically palliative effects of opium and its potential to ruin and destroy lives. Two bare lines from the early nineteenth-century playwright Joanna Baillie express this desolation:

6 Sir J. Hawkins, *The Life of Samuel Johnson 1719-1784* (1962), p.133.
7 Ibid.
8 R. Holmes, *Shelley: The Pursuit* (1994), pp.391-2.
9 Ibid., pp.111, 113.

Some opiate drug would be to him, I reckon,
Worth all my company, and something more.[10]

And the poem, 'TO ONE, who had taken laudanum to enliven himself' (1820), is another example of a piercing plea for the restoration of a loved one lost to opium:

And canst thou thus, my Edwin, woo thy doom
When there are those who prize thy life so dearly,
Because a transient gloom obscures thy soul,
And thy pulse beats not to its wonted time?
Mad pleasure's throb we may not always know:-
The heart's bright ruby streams would burst their bourns
And struggling life sink in the wild disorder ...

Or (can it please thee better?) lie thou long,
Wasted and languid on the late-sought couch.
And when the hour inert grows too oppressive,
Slowly arise enervate, and with hand
That trembling does its office, faintly reach
Th' infernal poppy's black and baleful juice.
The which I ne'er behold, but a cold corse
All grim with poison, from its bed impure
Rises distinct to fright my shrinking fancy ...

Thou guard against thy heart susceptible and learn
To love such calm delights as hide not death ...

And scorn not the remonstrance of a friend.[11]

Many addicts underwent great tribulations suffering from the oppressive enervation of a life devoted to opium. Sir Walter Scott made many attempts to do without the drug, believing it to be an 'immense point gained' if he could, for he recognised it as being extremely hurtful to his general health.[12] The chronic illnesses that Scott suffered had, by 1819, reduced him to 'the very image of Death ... lanthorn-jawed, decayed in flesh, stooping', and his distress and agony eventually lead him into addiction. But, worse than this, the analgesic effects he craved often eluded him utterly, perhaps because he attempted to curb his intake without taking into account his level of tolerance. 'Conceive my having taken', he wrote, 'in the course of six or seven hours, six grains of opium, three of hyoscamus, near twenty drops of laudanum – and all without any sensible relief of the agony under which I laboured

10 Joanna Baillie (1762-1851), 'The Phantom: A Musical Drama, in Two Acts' from *The Dramatic and Poetical Works* 'Miscellaneous Plays' (1851), Act II, Scene VI.

11 Maria Gowen Brooks, 'TO ONE, who had taken laudanum to enliven himself', from *Judith, Esther, and other poems* (1820).

12 J. Gibson Lockhart, *The Life of Sir Walter Scott* (1902), 6, pp.53-7.

... it has been a terrible set to'.[13] That same year, 1819, Scott's epic poem 'The Bride of Lammermoor' reached the printer who, from his own deathbed, later dictated the following account of the author's state:

> The book ... was not only written, but published, before Mr Scott was able to rise from his bed; and he assured me, that when it was first put into his hands in a complete shape, he did not recollect one single incident, character, or conversation it contained! ... not a single character woven by the romancer, not one of the many scenes and points of humour, nor anything with which he was connected as the writer of the work. "For a long time", he said, "I felt myself very uneasy in the course of my reading, lest I should be startled by reading something altogether glaring and fantastic ... as a whole, I felt it monstrous gross and grotesque; but still the worst of it made me laugh". I do not think I ever ventured to lead to the discussion of this singular phenomenon again; but you may depend upon it, that what I have said now is as distinctly reported as if it had been taken in short-hand at the moment ... I believe you will agree with me in thinking that the history of the human mind contains nothing more wonderful.[14]

Critics have argued that, after 1818, Scott produced more fantastic and mystical work than his earlier acclaimed contemporary realism and that the two genres did not compare well. But the intensely emotional character of the later work, probably influenced by his use of opium, has also been hailed for providing a 'new kind of truth about the human condition', a profound sensitivity that was previously lacking.[15]

Broad cultural images of female sensitivity, present in novels, drama, poetry, painting, popular ballads and opera, supported the idea of mentally and emotionally weak womanhood peculiarly susceptible to addiction.[16] Prone as she was seen to be to her emotions and to irrationality, given to reaction rather than initiation, there existed an underlying and persistently prejudicial assumption about the weakness of the female will, an idea exploited by physicians in terms of pathology, and which is addressed in chapter six.[17] The opium experiences of Dorothy Wordsworth show us some of the reasons how and why a woman might become addicted and how she might be treated by others, even by those with an intimate knowledge, themselves, of what addiction meant.

Dorothy was described by De Quincey as suffering from 'agitation of her excessive organic sensibility, and perhaps, from some morbid irritability of the nerves', and she had taken refuge in the mercies of laudanum. She too had begun a habit for want of relief from pain and sickness, firstly with severe toothache and then later for sick headaches, stomach cramps, lethargy and bowel disorder. The latter symptoms correspond with those of withdrawal from opium use and may have been such. Her letters and journal record her self-medication: she was sometimes 'ill in

---

13 Ibid.

14 Ibid., pp.63, 81-2.

15 Butler, *Romantics*, p.150.

16 A. Scull, *The Most Solitary of Afflictions: Madness and Society in Britain 1700-1900* (1993), p.159.

17 See also Oppenheim, *Shattered Nerves*, pp.181-232.

the afternoon, took laudanum' or 'took laudanum … lay in bed all day'. Mary, her sister-in-law, commented that Dorothy might maintain her health if she could 'be prevailed upon to abide by the plan of *abstinence* from several things, which will be hard for her to do'. But her husband believed that the opium was destroying her and that it contributed to an increasing dementia, despite her attempts to halve her dose. He wrote that he had 'always thought that this weakening of the mind has been caused by the opium which was thought necessary on account of her great bodily sufferings'. Though he saw her in a 'sad state when the action of the opium is not upon her' he confessed that 'I feel my hand shaking, I have had so much agitation today, in attempting to quiet my poor Sister, and from being under the necessity of refusing her things that would be improper for her'. Dorothy's habit was at all times the province of her family and she was submissive to their ministrations and demands.

During the 1830s her family began a regime to wean her off her opium. They wrote to friends asking that they stay away as 'it would add to our distress if you should be a witness of the anxiety we are undergoing on account of the experiment now in progress, and drawing towards a conclusion' and 'we would rather you were not conscious of them to the extent that would be unavoidable if you were with us'. Though they believed that the opium was necessary for her in some ways and though 'her present sufferings … from withdrawing this medicine [were] so severe' they still expected 'in the course of a fortnight to get rid of it altogether'. The experiment was a disappointment and Dorothy and her family continued to live with her habit, and her degenerating mental health, until her death at eighty-four; a long life despite, or perhaps because of, the opium.[18]

Coleridge's daughter Sara, an insomniac, began addiction to opium in 1825 for the precious sleep it gave her. She became ever more enraptured following the births of her children in 1830 and 1832, both events having been attended throughout by Gillman, the physician who had supervised her father's opium habit. Gillman diagnosed 'nervous debility' and prescribed her laudanum. She had thought it a '*horrid* drug' when used by her father or De Quincey, but for herself she thought this label 'rather ungrateful as it has done me much good and no harm'. She revealed to a friend that she was 'unable to sleep at all without laudanum, which I regret much', but still she believed that, despite knowledge of her father's habit, she would not 'find any difficulty in leaving it off'. Sara's description of herself as a 'creature doomed to despair' did not persuade her husband to grant her a respite from childbirth and she fell again, this time for twins, in 1833. The babies both died within a few days of their traumatic birth and six months later the bereaved young mother suffered the additional loss of her father. Barely eating, taking little except opium, she became malnourished and amenorrhoetic, which at least prevented further pregnancies. As she increased her doses of opium she acknowledged her habit publicly in a poem from her volume *Pretty Lessons in Verse* (1834). Members of the Coleridge family rued its inclusion and Sara herself, mindful of her father's infamous reputation,

18 Jones, *Passionate Sisterhood*, pp.178, 268-70, 285.

and shamed by any reflection on the family, agreed that 'the Poppy poem in *Pretty Lessons* should have been left out', though it remained in subsequent editions.[19] It speaks of innocence and experience:

> The Poppies Blooming all around
> My Herbert loves to see,
> Some pearly white, some dark as night,
> Some red as cramasie;
>
> He loves their colours fresh and fine
> As fair as fair may be,
> But little does my darling know
> How good they are to me.
>
> He views their clustering petals gay
> And shakes their nut-brown seeds.
> But they to him are nothing more
> Than other brilliant weeds;
>
> O how should'st thou with beaming brow
> With eye and cheek so bright
> Know aught of that blossom's pow'r,
> Or sorrows of the night!
>
> When poor mama long restless lies
> She drinks the poppy's juice;
> That liquor soon can close her eyes
> And slumber soft produce.
>
> O' then my sweet my happy boy
> Will thank the poppy flow'r
> Which brings the sleep to dear mama
> At midnight's darksome hour.[20]

Many literary figures of the eighteenth and nineteenth centuries indulged in opium. De Quincey and Coleridge were not exceptional, except in the degree of their use. Fanny Trollope, for example, in late middle-age, established a routine of writing her books by night, 'helped by laudanum and green tea'. Harriet Martineau, recalling the 1830s and 40s, claimed that a clergyman who knew the literary world well, had informed her that 'there was no author or authoress who was free from the habit of taking some pernicious stimulant; either … wine or spirits or laudanum'. The amount of opium taken to relieve the mental and physical travails of creativity was,

19 Ibid., pp.271-5, 280-3.

20 Ibid.

he maintained, 'greater than most people had any conception of, and all literary workers took something'.[21]

Elizabeth Barrett Browning and Robert Browning

How sad and bad and mad it was - But then, how it was sweet

Robert Browning, *Confessions*

A deep poignancy lies within this confessional phrase of Robert Browning's. And yet more besides, for the poet unerringly answers the question: why give yourself over to enslavement? Why, he rhetorically answers, but for the sensation of being embraced by a pleasure that is worth the depredations of any risks involved, even social vilification. Whilst he spoke of self-abandonment to pleasure, he led one to feel that it might be the very sadness, badness and madness of enslavement that rendered it at once so sweet and so bitter a condition. Without sensation how else would one know one was alive? And in the very act of experiencing and recording one's own 'living', one knowingly tempts one's own demise. A poignant, paradoxical self-poisoning.

In the 1840s Elizabeth Barrett Browning wrote to her husband asking, 'Can I be as good for you as morphine is for me, I wonder, even at the cost of being as bad also? – Can't you leave me off without risking your life, - nor go on with me without running all the hazards of poison - ?' And he, taking up the intimate analogy, in turn asked her 'May I call you my morphine?' and enquired of her how she could ever imagine he might continue 'without my proper quantity' of the metaphorical drug.[22]

Elizabeth had been reliant on opium since the age of fourteen. Her physicians had prescribed the drug when she was afflicted with a mysterious idiopathic ailment, opaquely described as a 'derangement in some highly important organ'. As the most effectively pervasive and calming medicine in the pharmacopoeia there was little choice of treatment given the obscure and puzzling symptoms she displayed. In 1846 Robert expressed his concerns about Elizabeth's habitual use of opium and provoked a gently surprised reaction. She answered, 'that you should care so much about the opium -! Then *I* must care, & get to do with less … at least'. The drug had become as much a part of her daily existence as food and drink, but she understood that it might seem strange, worrisome and distasteful to others. In the same letter she explained to her husband that she needed 'opium in any shape' to relieve her distressing physical symptoms. Describing these she wrote: 'I have had a restlessness till it made me almost mad – at one time I lost the power of sleeping quite … as if one's life, instead

21 Except, of course, Miss Martineau. V. Glendinning, *Trollope* (1993), p.63.

22 J. Markus, *Dared and Done: The Marriage of Elizabeth Barrett and Robert Browning* (1995), p.51.

of giving movement to the body, were imprisoned and diminished within it, & beating and fluttering impatiently to get out, at all the doors & windows'.[23]

For this agitation, which sounds very much like withdrawal, the physiological response to the absence of the drug, rather than any illness, her doctors prescribed more opium. 'A preparation of it', as she reported, 'called morphine ... & ever since I have been calling it ... my elixir ... the tranquillizing power has been so wonderful'. Elizabeth was very aware of possible condemnation of her habitual drug use and wanted her husband to understand that she 'never *increased* upon the prescribed quantity ... no! – now think of my writing all this to you!' The opium, she assured him, was used to 'balance the nervous system' and was not taken for her 'spirits' in the 'usual sense'. She was anxious that he 'must not think such a thing'.[24] Describing the luxurious or, as it were, uplifting use of opium as being 'usual', Elizabeth betrayed an easy and quite blasé appreciation of its attractions. She also understood that this behaviour might be frowned upon as degenerate and consequently was at pains to emphasise her own use of the drug as medicinal and therefore respectable. This manipulative explanation and self-justification fits well with what has been described as 'society's perennially ambiguous attitudes towards the sick' in that it allowed her some sympathetic leeway and a 'legitimate deviance', something ideally suited to, and coveted by, the habitual user of opium.[25]

Elizabeth did not seriously attempt to reduce her dependence on the drug until she entered her forties, when she 'gradually diminish[ed] the dose to seventeen days for twenty-two doses which I used to take in eight days'. This self-inflicted withdrawal was inspired by the first of two miscarriages and the fear that the drug may have poisoned and destroyed the child. She continued her regime of abstinence, showing, her husband believed, 'extraordinary strength equal to that of a thousand men', and she gave birth to a son in 1849 at the age of forty-three.[26]

By the late 1850s Elizabeth's use of opium was again an issue between husband and wife and was also becoming increasingly public knowledge, particularly following the emotional blow she suffered at the death of her father. There was gossip, some of it malicious, and some of it finding its way into print. The American poet, Julia Ward Howe, author of, among other works, 'The Battle Hymn of the Republic', having

23 Ibid.

24 Ibid., p.40

25 R. Porter, ed., *The Cambridge Illustrated History of Medicine* (1996), p.111. The idea of 'legitimate deviance' originated with the work of the American sociologist Talcott Parsons in the 1950s. He regarded the 'sick role', even the '*malade imaginaire*', as a 'tacit deal between sufferers and society' which allowed one to be temporarily relieved of social responsibilities. See also E. Shorter, *From Paralysis to Fatigue: A History of Psychosomatic Illness in the Modern Era* (1992), chapter 1, wherein the author discusses a vast range of nervous symptoms and eccentricities and sees them as emanating from 'codes' or 'rules' of behaviour governing the sick which are propagated by physicians and unconsciously adhered to by patients.

26 Markus, *Dared and Done*, pp.90, 130.

been slighted by Elizabeth, published a volume in 1857 containing a spiteful piece entitled 'One word more with E.B.B'. It ran as follows:

> I shrink before the nameless draught
> That help to such unearthly things,
> And if a drug could lift so high,
> I would not trust its treacherous wings;
>
> Lest, leaping from them, I should fall,
> A weight more dead than stock or stone, -
> The warning fate of those who fly
> With pinions other than their own.[27]

Robert Browning's feelings of outrage on behalf of his wife at this very public attack, presumably also based on a sense of exposure and shame, were not shared by Elizabeth. She placated him, telling him that she was 'not a bit' angry, that the poem had referred to a 'nameless drug', and that indeed, the thing was 'perfectly true, so far, that life is necessary to writing, & that I should not be alive except by help of my morphine'.[28] Elizabeth might have been content to tell the truth and shame the devil but Robert was repelled by the idea of her habit becoming a subject for public gossip, for to be exposed was to be unprotected and to invite ridicule and contempt. How ambivalent he must have felt about the opium, and how his own feelings mirrored society's dichotomous attitudes towards its uses. Janus-faced, the drug offered both succour and destruction. As a medicine it was indispensable and thaumaturgic; as a poison it was ruinous, shameful and sometimes ultimately fatal.

Lizzie Siddall and Dante Gabriel Rossetti

The poet Lizzie Siddall, muse and eventually wife to the Pre-Raphaelite painter Dante Gabriel Rossetti, was also an habitual laudanum drinker, an addict who died of the effects of the drug, though in less than clear circumstances. She had endured great disappointment and emotional cruelty at Rossetti's hands and had suffered for many years from what was probably a psychosomatic illness. Certainly her circumstances had not matched her expectations and her physicians were hard put to diagnose her symptoms. Unable to eat properly, she vomited up any useful sustenance for weeks at a time and spent months in her bed, for long periods too weak to move. Rossetti, despite his often reprehensible behaviour, was nonetheless deeply moved by Lizzie's plight, and had his patron, John Ruskin, arrange for her to see the eminent London physician, Henry Acland. The 'leading cause' of her illness, Acland believed, was the result of 'the strain under which she had been living'. During the 1850s one of her physicians prescribed laudanum to calm her nerves and her stomach pains and, by her own admission, she became addicted, drinking 'quarts' of the tincture over

---

27 Ibid.
28 Ibid., pp.277-8.

the coming years. She recorded her experiences of a racing pulse, chills, fevers and violent fits of trembling whenever she had to do without her drug. Lizzie's continuing illness and misery, compounded by the loss of a child, robbed her of any resilience she had had. She wrote her last poem, 'Lord, May I Come?', in a hand described by Rossetti as 'shaky and straggling', and he thought that 'it must have been done under the influence of laudanum, which she frequently took by medical orders as a palliative'.[29]

On the night of 10 February 1862 Rossetti discovered Lizzie in a deeply stupefied state, an empty laudanum bottle on her bedside stand. A physician, Francis Hutchinson, was immediately summoned but, despite the use of a stomach pump and the assistance of a second doctor, she died seven hours later. At her inquest the following day Rossetti told the coroner of her habitual use of laudanum. He knew, he said, 'that she had taken a hundred drops', but he did not think she had intended to kill herself that night. He told the court that she took the drug 'to quiet her nerves', and that 'she could not have lived without laudanum'. Her physician gave it as his opinion that she had taken 'a very large dose' after suffering terribly during her pregnancy. She had been forced to carry the child dead in her belly for two weeks before its birth. The jury found that Lizzie had 'accidentally, casually, and by misfortune [come] to her death'. Nonetheless, stories and rumour abounded. Some had it that she had been murdered, poisoned, by Rossetti, and tales of his cruel behaviour towards her were repeated as evidence. Oscar Wilde postulated that the infuriated artist had pressed the poison into her hands, shouting at her to 'take the lot', before storming out of the house. But most of those close to Lizzie believed she had deliberately taken her life in despair. Her husband later attempted suicide with laudanum himself and, though he was resuscitated with inhalations of ammonia and draughts of strong coffee, he suffered partial paralysis for some time afterwards.[30]

Rossetti's death at the age of fifty-three in 1881, has been described as 'a denouement induced altogether by narcotism which has no respect for person or genius and makes slaves of the most exalted men'.[31] Edmund Gosse, however, a contemporary of Rossetti's, gave his friend a more gracious and less judgemental obituary writing that 'his mighty spirit was an outlaw yet in this bright garish modern life of ours', and he was relieved that the world had ceased 'to vex him with her wasting care'.[32] Rossetti's known drugs of choice were alcohol, chloral and opium.[33]

29 G. Daly, *Pre-Raphaelites in Love* (1989), chapter 2; Berridge and Edwards, *Opium*, p.80; Macht and Gessford, 'The Unfortunate Drug Experiences of Dante Gabriel Rossetti', *Institute of the History of Medicine Bulletin*, 1938, 6, pp.34-61.

30 Ibid.

31 Macht and Gessford, *The Unfortunate Drug Experiences*, p.35.

32 Edmund Gosse, 'Dante Gabriel Rossetti' (1882), in *In Russet & Silver. Miscellaneous Poems* (1894), pp.99-101, lines 19, 20, 42.

33 Chloral Hydrate was developed in 1832 by the chemist Liebig who also was instrumental in the introduction of Chloroform. Chloral, however, a soporific and hypnotic, was not used generally until the 1860s, and its rapid action marked it out as a potentially dangerous drug.

He was introduced to chloral in the 1870s by an intimate friend, the painter, journalist and American Consul, William J. Stillman, who recounted that Rossetti was:

> sleepless, excitable, and possessed by the monomania of persecution … I recommended him to try chloral, then a nearly new remedy which I had used by prescription with excellent effect for my own sleeplessness, and which I always carried with me. I gave him twenty grains dissolved in water to be taken at three doses. But, as he forgot it on the first two nights, he took the whole on the third (twenty grains) … at a subsequent time, taking it on the prescription of a physician, he fell into the habit of using it to his great injury, from the want of self control in the employment of it.[34]

Stillman also recommended the 'splendid sleeping potion' to Ford Maddox Brown in 1868, and his son Oliver suggested the following regime to a friend in 1870:

> A dose of *Chloral* on Monday, *Sour Milk* on Tuesday, *Laudanum* on Wednesdays, on Thursday a little *Spirits* … while on Friday you might modestly content yourself with fifteen to twenty five drops of *Chlorodyne*. In this way you would not grow hardened to any one of them, and each would retain its full power and proper efficiency.[35]

Rossetti's brother, William, saw Stillman and his 'friendly ministrations' as 'a remedy worse than the disease'. His brother was a man 'least fitted to try such an experiment with impunity', and, with his particular temperament, it was 'a case of any expedient, and any risk to escape a present evil'. Dante Rossetti began with nightly doses of ten grains which, in time, were increased to a hundred and eighty grains, though his physician, 'knowing with whom he had to deal', ordered the chemist to begin secretly diluting the mixture. Even so it was thought that 'no case has been recorded in the annals of medicine in which one patient has taken so much or even half so much chloral as Rossetti took'. In fact, by November 1879, the chemists Messrs Bell & Company, had refused to allow him more than one bottle a day rather than the dozen he had been receiving every week or so.[36] His 'chloralism' was treated with morphine, and the fine cocktail of substances which Rossetti daily imbibed was recorded by one of his attending physicians in his last months when detailing the artist's great agitation and 'craving' for whiskey, chloral, ether, brandy, morphine and laudanum.[37] The last was a familiar drug for Rossetti, one that he had attempted suicide with and which, his brother believed, he may have 'long had about him … even before he began the nightly course of chloral'.

---

34 Macht and Gessford, *The Unfortunate Drug Experiences*, p.53.
35 Ibid.
36 Ibid., pp.37-8.
37 Ibid., p.40.

Opium addiction in mid- to late Victorian fiction

Similar experiences and accounts of opium use crept constantly to and fro between reality and fiction during the nineteenth century, providing a public forum for the airing and forming of attitudes towards them. A pleasurable gathering of characters in Anne Brontë's *Tenant of Wildfell Hall* (1848), for example, discussed the 'hankering after forbidden things' and the 'evils' of intemperance and abstinence: being the central Victorian questions of the voluntary nature of the Will, and of indulgence and self-denial. Suggesting that, whilst it might be prudent to allow a child a taste of forbidden substances to remove any sense of a dangerous mystique, they agree amongst themselves that 'most of us had better abstain from [laudanum], even in moderation'. This is despite the acknowledgement that it is still generally and 'rightly' regarded as a 'blessing of Providence'.[38]

Brontë followed this argument with a moral example illustrating the dangerous pitfalls she saw inherent in unorthodox opium use. She introduced the debauched character Arthur Huntingdon, who is made partially responsible for the corruption and degradation of Lord Lowborough. The weak-willed Lowborough, finally attempting to forsake the 'rank poison' of alcohol, resorts to another poison, a 'private bottle of laudanum … which he was continually soaking at – or rather, holding off and on with, abstaining one day, and exceeding the next – just like the spirits'. Eventually this ruined character becomes an unreliable attendee of his friend's 'orgies', gliding in like a 'spectre' or 'the ghost from Macbeth', sitting silently in a corner, 'suffering from an overdose of his insidious comforter'. Occasionally the unfortunate wretch would startle the company with an impassioned outburst: 'What you see in life I don't know – I see only the blackness of darkness, and a fearful looking for of judgement and fiery indignation!' His companion's response was to simply bid him drink with them and 'he would soon see as bright a prospect as any [of them]'.[39] They were unburdened of conscience or forethought by their indulgences, and existed in a destructive, short-lived, luxurious present.

Anne Brontë relied on her personal knowledge of opium-taking for these characterisations and arguments. Aside from the correspondence that ran between the Brontë family and De Quincey, Anne's brother, Branwell, was a gin-drinker and confirmed laudanum addict.[40] He was also, most probably, her model for Lowborough, whose 'little store of gin and laudanum' brought him 'blessed release' from mental pain and misery. She was able to describe the 'blotting out of feeling' that Branwell craved, and the feelings he experienced 'before full oblivion set in' of 'such strange and wandering images [that] filled the room'. Their sister Charlotte, writing to her friend Ellen Nussey on 3 March 1846, confided that 'it was very forced work to address [Branwell]. I might have spared myself the trouble, as he took no notice, and made no reply; he was stupefied'. She wrote that her 'fears

38 Anne Brontë, *The Tenant of Wildfell Hall* (1848), p.37.

39 Ibid., pp.160-1.

40 Lindop, *The Opium-Eater*, p.339.

were not vain', and that Emily Brontë had admitted that 'he got a sovereign from Papa while I have been away, under the pretence of paying a passing debt … and has employed it as was to be expected'. His sisters felt Branwell to be a 'hopeless being' and that at times it was 'scarcely possible to stay in the room where he is'. They despaired of his future. And, in fact, after a self-acknowledged disappointed life, he died in debt and duplicity, aged 31 years.[41] His friend, Francis Grundy, wrote of Branwell that he 'was no domestic demon – he was just a man moving in a mist who lost his way … *at least* he proved the reality of his sorrows'.[42] But the whole of the family had struggled with the addiction and had lived through frightening and demoralising incidences: candles were upset; bedclothes caught fire; carving knives were concealed; and lies told.[43]

The senses of alienation, of disruptive transformation and of a mirror-like view of respectable society are ideas and circumstances exploited by Charles Dickens throughout his fictional works. A worn down underclass of opium-eating proletariat inhabits the fictional Coketown of *Hard Times* (1854): the chemist and druggist, 'with other tabular statements, showing that when they didn't get drunk, they took opium'.[44] In *Bleak House* (1853) the lawyer, Mr Tulkinghorn, discovers the cadaver of a solitary forsaken man, known only as *Nemo*, who has died of an opium overdose.[45] Entering the 'foul and filthy room' where the body lies 'there comes into the lawyer's mouth the bitter, vapid taste of opium' and there is enough left by the bed to kill a dozen people. Those gathered in the aftermath of this sordid death are strangers to each other and to the dead man, emphasising the sense of alienation and futility. He has no identity other than that of an opium addict. The landlord is ignorant of his deceased tenant, the surgeon who had sold him his opium for the last year and a half knew him only by sight, yet speculates that it is not a suicide as 'he has been in the habit of taking so much'. This is all there is to be said about the 'man unknown' and, after a cursory inquest the coroner returns a verdict of accidental death: 'No doubt. Gentleman you are discharged. Good afternoon.' From a mean and pitiful life and death the unknown man is 'sown in corruption' in a 'hemmed-in churchyard, pestiferous and obscene'.[46]

Dickens based Esther's *Bleak House* narrative of illness and dreams on passages from De Quincey's *Confessions*, and he used the work again in his unfinished novel, *The Mystery of Edwin Drood* (1870).[47] Echoing De Quincey's autobiographical account of his search for Anne in and around the alleys that led off the central thoroughfare of Oxford Street, Dickens's opium-addicted, anti-hero John Jasper, embodying the seemingly antithetical roles of choirmaster and murderer, searches

41 J. Barker, *The Brontës* (1994), pp.512-516.
42 Ibid., p.569.
43 D. Du Maurier, *The Infernal World of Branwell Brontë* (1960), pp.181, 183.
44 Dickens, *Hard Times* (1854), p.66.
45 S. Shatto, *The Companion to Bleak House* (1988), p.107.
46 Dickens, *Bleak House* (1853), chapter 11, pp.125-37.
47 Shatto, *Companion to Bleak House*, p.220.

for the illusory character of his dreams in Dickens's familiar domain: the depths of the urban labyrinth.[48] For the relevant scenes in *Edwin Drood* Dickens himself made accompanied forays in the late 1860s to the 'out-of-the-way' sights of London. The Hon. Frederick Wellesley recorded that, between 1863 and 1866, they followed the current fashion of 'doing the slums' and went on nocturnal visits to the city's opium dens in and around Shadwell. Dickens's small group consisted of a policeman, Charley Field, who was nominated by the Chief Commissioner of Police and was the original of Inspector Bucket in *Bleak House*, and his friends George Dolby, Sol Eytinge, and J.T. Fields.[49] In a miserable court at night they came across 'a haggard old woman blowing at a kind of pipe made of an old ink bottle', an image which anticipates the experiences of Doré and Jerrold in *London: A Pilgrimage* (1872). Fields recounted that 'the identical words which Dickens puts into the mouth of this wretched creature in *Edwin Drood* we heard her croon as we leaned over the tattered bed in which she was lying ... and the Chinamen and Lascars made never-to-be-forgotten pictures in the scene'.[50] The haggard woman makes fictitious parodied appearances in the novel as 'Er Royal Highness the Princess Puffer' and the 'Hopeum Puffer', but the original of the character was probably one 'Lascar Sal', or 'Sally the opium-eater', who was well known to the Metropolitan Police and the slumming swells. According to Wellesley who met her during the years 1863-66 she was in her mid-twenties but, in his opinion, appeared physically to be a much older woman, worn down by her opium habit and other deprivations.[51] Opium was associated with a world of excess and degradation in Dickens's novels. It is a potentially ruinous element in otherwise good and productive lives or it is a symbol of inherent evil. But it is known that, like many others, Dickens saw another side to the drug, for he himself took laudanum to ease pain and illness, and he also used it to calm himself and induce sleep when on his reading tour of America in 1867-68.

Dickens was a great friend of the novelist Wilkie Collins, with whom he no doubt discussed the effects of narcosis. And Collins was a great admirer of 'The Bride of Lammermoor', he knew that Scott had taken laudanum during the writing of it, and he had collected accounts of writers with an opium habit.[52] He himself became an *habitué* during his productive literary adult life, his mother was Coleridge's 'exceedingly sensible woman', and his father's last chronic illness was alleviated by 'Batley's Drops', a popular proprietary opiate.

In 1868, when he was in his thirties, Collins succumbed to a painful rheumatic illness, was reduced to complete prostration by the death of his mother, and came to rely heavily on the physical and mental analgesic effects of opium. He completed

---

48 L. Frank, *Charles Dickens and the Romantic Self* (1984), p.189.

49 P. Collins, 'Inspector Bucket Visits The Princess Puffer', *The Dickensian*, January 1964, 60, no. 342, pp.88-90.

50 G. Gissing, ed., *Forster's Life of Dickens* (1903), pp.305-7.

51 Dickens, *The Mystery of Edwin Drood* (1870), p.314, n.4; Collins, 'Inspector Bucket Visits The Princess Puffer', p.90.

52 Hayter, *Opium and the Romantic Imagination*, p.294.

The Moonstone during this period, dictating it from his bed, according to his own account, in remarkably similar circumstances to those in which Scott had written 'The Bride of Lammermoor'. A secretary was found who 'wrote on steadily in spite of my cries [and] when it was finished I was not only pleased and astonished at the finale, but did not recognise it as my own'.[53]

Twenty years later, in agreement with contemporary medical opinion with which he was obviously very familiar, Collins was extolling the stimulating effects of opium upon the brain and its soothing effects upon the nerves, and he recommended it to his friends. To one who had tried it and been less enthusiastic he wrote:

> Your report is disappointing to your medical adviser … Laudanum has a two fold action on the brain and nervous system – a stimulating and a sedative action. It seems but *too* plain to me that *your* nerves are so strongly affected by the stimulating action that they are incapable of feeling the sedative action which ought to follow. Whether a considerably larger dose than any you have taken would have the right effect I dare not ask. Such a risk is not to be run except under a competent medical adviser.[54]

Much of Collins's work was produced in a state of 'nervous concentration', and, again in agreement with medical theory on nervous diseases, believed that there was no fatigue equal to that which 'comes of daily working of the brains for hours together'.[55] This being an accepted scientific truism, it was also thought, as will become clear in Part II, that addiction was a symptom of such heightened sensibilities. Collins was a model opium addict.

His doses of opium were considered quite heroic, and, in the opinion of the eminent surgeon Sir William Fergusson, who was dining with him one evening, his nightly dose alone was sufficient to kill everyone round the table. A servant in the household had in fact already died after having taken only half the wine glass full of laudanum that Collins had poured for himself. His friends were often called upon to help him procure opium if he was indisposed or in difficulties. On a tour of Switzerland he had sought help when his supply had run out, 'I am in terrible trouble', he wrote in a note to his companion,

> I know, however, that there are six chemists at Coire; and if you and I pretend, separately, to be physicians, and each chemist consents to give each of us the maximum of opium he may by Swiss law, which is very strict, give to one person, I shall just have enough to get through the night … if we fail, heaven help me![56]

He took some comfort, though, from the thought that his habit was not comparable to that of De Quincey, who had quaffed his laudanum from a jug.[57]

53 W.M. Clarke, *The Secret Life of Wilkie Collins* (1988), pp.113-14.

54 Ibid., p.165.

55 Ibid., pp. 162-3.

56 Ibid., p.164.

57 J. Symons, 'Introduction' to Wilkie Collins, *The Woman in White* (1860), p.9.

Opium became Collins's 'only friend', and though he often declared he could control his habit despite his heroic doses, he had made his first attempt to wean himself off of it under his physician's instructions in 1869. In a candid letter to a friend he confided that he was being 'stabbed every night at ten, with a sharp-pointed syringe which injects morphia under my skin ... without any of the drawbacks of taking opium internally'. His was assured that if he persevered he would eventually be able to diminish the dose of morphia and 'so emancipate [himself] from opium altogether', a goal which he never realised.[58] Hall Caine recounted a conversation with the novelist who, declaring he would show his friend 'the secrets of my prison-house', confided that he had taken laudanum for twenty years 'to stimulate the brain and steady the nerves'. And, Collins said, he knew of other writers who took it for the same purposes, Bulwer Lytton for one, had told him this himself. But Hall Caine also maintained that when he asked his friend whether he would recommend it to him for his nervous exhaustion, Collins 'paused, changed colour slightly, and then said quietly "No"'.[59]

'Darling' opium infused the intricate plots of Collins's novels. The heroine of *No Name* (1862) clutches her laudanum and considers suicide whilst that of *Armadale* (1866) takes it as a restorative for her nerves. She cries, 'who was the man who invented laudanum? I thank him from the bottom of my heart ... if all the miserable wretches in pain of body and mind, whose comforter he has been, could meet together to sing his praises, what a chorus it would be!'[60] The plot of *The Moonstone* (1868) rests on the mercurial powers of opium, where the drug simultaneously provides and obscures the central mystery and where it is both feared and welcomed by those who use it. The character of Ezra Jennings, narrator, medical man, and arguably, for his opium experiences, an autobiographical creation, is compelled to submit to 'the vengeance' and frightful dreams of a regular 500 drops of laudanum to quell the pain of a chronic 'internal complaint'. It is the 'one effective palliative ... all-potent, all merciful drug' and Jennings considers himself to be 'indebted to a respite of many years from a sentence of death'. But he is trapped by its mercy, for 'even the virtues of opium have their limit' and the progress of his disease has gradually forced him 'from the use of opium, to the abuse of it'. He feels the 'penalty' at last, his 'nervous system is shattered [his] nights are nights of horror' and he fearfully anticipates his impending death. Despite his own experiences, Jennings is paradoxically experimenting with the drug on someone else in order to reveal reality and truth for the benefit and advantage of others. The contradictions and the idiosyncratic effects of opium are faithfully recorded in the novel, and it is remarked at one point that it is a truism that 'there are probably no two men in existence on whom the drug acts

58 Hayter, *Opium and the Romantic Imagination*, p.294; Clarke, *Secret Life of Wilkie Collins*, pp.121-2.

59 Hayter, *Opium and the Romantic Imagination*, p.294.

60 Ibid.

in exactly the same manner'. And what anyway, the omniscient voice of the author asks, 'is experience where opium is concerned?'[61]

The resourceful Mr Christian in Eliot's *Felix Holt* (1866) was a captive of opium who also suffered from an 'access of nervous pains', and he 'did what he could: he took doses of opium'. But he 'consoled himself as to future possibilities' with the thought that, if the pains ever became too frequent or intolerable, a simple increase in the dose would put an end to them altogether.[62] Eliot gave this melancholy end to the abandoned and destitute character Molly in *Silas Marner* (1861). Molly, with her small daughter, is reduced to vagrancy and has sunk to finding solace in 'draughts of forgetfulness'. But the neglect she has suffered, though appalling enough, is not reason enough for her condition: it is 'the demon Opium to whom she was enslaved, body and soul' that has brought her so low. She must bear responsibility for herself in that respect and, 'in the moments of unbenumbed consciousness', she recognises 'her want and degradation' as partially self-inflicted. She needed comfort and 'knew but one comforter – the familiar demon in her bosom ... the black remnant' that gave her the 'complete torpor ... at last'.[63] Eliot's audience were far from unaccustomed to stories of ruin such as these; they read them almost daily in the press, as we will see, and they read into them attitudes of morality, destiny and tragedy.

Dr Lydgate, Eliot's idealistic young surgeon in *Middlemarch* (1871-72), becomes an opium user, though infrequently and then only under 'pressure of foreseen difficulties'. The doctor is a common fictional figure but here Eliot uses him to represent an emerging and new *type* of doctor, one who challenges the traditional order of the profession, and who inspires a great deal of animosity amongst his more hidebound colleagues. This professional resistance and hostility, together with the perception that his marriage has become virtually loveless, leads Lydgate to the balm of opium. But these episodes are sympathetically described as being merely the 'transient escapes from the hauntings of misery' of an otherwise good and worthy man, for the doctor had 'no hereditary constitutional cravings'.[64] Another *Middlemarch* character, the artist and romantic Will Ladislaw, who makes 'himself ill with doses of opium', *is* represented as decadent. He takes opium for gain, he aspires to genius, believes he 'must have the utmost play for its spontaneity', and that he should be 'placed in an attitude of receptivity' that would 'evolve the genius ... not yet come'. Unfortunately he, like many before him, is misguided and he discovers that there is a 'dissimilarity between his constitution and De Quincey's' for 'nothing greatly original had resulted from these measures'.[65] Yet another Eliotic artist admits to his friend that he has been smoking opium, having 'meant to do it sometime or

61 Wilkie Collins, *The Moonstone: A Romance* (1868), pp.135, 393, 405, 420.

62 George Eliot, *Felix Holt* (1866), p.233.

63 Eliot, *Silas Marner* (1861), p.155.

64 Eliot, *Middlemarch* (1871-72), p.720; see also B. Milligan, *Pleasures and Pains: Opium and the Orient in Nineteenth-Century British Culture* (1995), p.37. The question of a link between heredity and addiction is discussed in chapters 6 and 7.

65 Eliot, *Middlemarch*, p.109.

other', as if it had become a recognised rite of passage for the romantically inclined young man. Hans Meyrick, in *Daniel Deronda* (1876), when asked if he has been to Cambridge, replies that he has actually been to 'I-don't-know-where' under the influence of opium, to 'try how much bliss could be got by it'. But, like Ladislaw, he too suffers and is disappointed.[66]

Experience of unorthodox drug use also seeped from reality into the fiction of Sir Arthur Conan Doyle. He is said to have based the character of Sherlock Holmes on the eminent physician Joseph Bell, under whom he had studied medicine at Edinburgh. As a young man in the early 1880s, Conan Doyle made voyages to the Arctic and to Africa as a ship's doctor before joining the medical practice of a Dr Budd in Portsmouth. Budd died young, convinced he was being poisoned and eventually was driven to the extreme lengths of chemically testing every morsel of food set before him. Perhaps it was this and Budd's alleged lavish use of drugs that disturbed Conan Doyle and provoked him into leaving and setting up his own practice, first in Southsea and later in Devonshire Place, London, and to begin his prolific writing career.[67] It has been suggested that cocaine was chosen as Sherlock Holmes's favoured drug because of its novelty, and that even though the detective-aesthete also used opium, this was regarded in the 1890s as too quotidian a drug lacking the necessary exoticism which might set the user above the mediocre masses.[68] But, in *The Sign of Four* (1887), Holmes uses each drug according to his needs, causing the anxious and disapproving Dr Watson to ask fretfully, 'What is it today, morphine or cocaine?' Though he 'craves mental exaltation', Holmes can achieve this state through work and is then able to leave off his 'artificial stimulants', thereby controlling his intake. Nonetheless, Conan Doyle alludes to the dangers of addiction as he has Holmes ruminatively eyeing his 'sinewy forearm and wrist, all dotted and scarred with innumerable puncture marks' before he thrust 'the sharp point home, pressed down the tiny piston and sank back into the velvet armchair with a long sigh of satisfaction'.[69] In the short story 'The Man with the Twisted Lip' (1891), Holmes visits an opium den in a 'vile alley' in the 'furthest' East End docklands of London, a haunt replete with the usual suspects, the Lascars and Malays, muttering and mumbling in their drugged isolation. The den also shrouds a respectable but fallen friend of Watson's, 'much addicted to opium', whose habit had grown upon him after he had soaked his tobacco with laudanum in an attempt to experience 'De Quincey's description of his dreams and sensations'. He had been gradually reduced to a 'wreck and ruin of a noble man', with the ubiquitous 'yellow, pasty face, drooping lids and pin-point pupils, all huddled in a chair'.[70]

---

66 Eliot, *Daniel Deronda* (1876), p.853.

67 J. Symons, *Portrait of an Artist: Conan Doyle* (1979), pp.42, 45.

68 R. Pearsall, *Conan Doyle: A Biographical Solution* (1977), pp.55-6.

69 Arthur Conan Doyle 'The Sign of Four' (1887) in *The Original Illustrated 'Strand' Sherlock Holmes* (1998), p.64.

70 'The Man with the Twisted Lip', Ibid., p.186.

Corruption, contamination, and degeneration are heavily present, too, in Oscar Wilde's *The Picture of Dorian Grey* (1891). The book was written following an evening spent with Conan Doyle, during which the two promised each other to write books for *Lippincott's Magazine*. Wilde produced *Dorian Grey*, and Conan Doyle *The Sign of Four*.[71] Opium has a terrible part to play in the hero's excessive and ruinous amoral behaviour. Dorian Grey, a *fin-de-siècle* icon of decadence, attempting to drive the knowledge of his accumulating crimes out of his conscious mind, must 'be drugged with poppies' to 'cure the soul by means of the senses'. Thus he ventures into opium dens 'where one could buy oblivion ... where memories of old sins could be destroyed by the madness of sins that were new', and where the 'hideous hunger for opium began to gnaw at him'. Malays are there in the den with him, 'showing their white teeth as they chattered', simian-like, and he encounters a lost friend among the inhuman 'grotesque things that lay in such fantastic postures on the ragged mattresses'. Grey is assured that 'as long as one has this stuff, one doesn't want friends'.[72] He and the reader discover for themselves the overwhelming and isolating potential of opium. Despite critical condemnation of its content, Conan Doyle thought *Dorian Grey* was 'surely [set] upon a high moral plane', and Wilde himself wrote that he could not 'understand how they can treat [it] as immoral ... the moral is too obvious'.[73]

Wilde gave short shrift to those who abused opium, a position illustrated by his comments made to his friend Sherard about the addiction of Maurice Rollinat in the 1880s. Rollinat was known as a 'talented poet and tragedian, an inspired musician, a marvellous artist' who refused to believe in progress, despairing instead of the 'stagnation of human perversity'. He took opium because he considered, in the Romantic tradition, that 'dreams and the fantastic' were necessary to his creative life. When Sherard, anxious about his response to Rollinat's self-destructive behaviour, analogously inquired of Wilde whether, if he saw a man throw himself into the river, he would not go after him. Wilde replied with chilling flippancy that he would 'consider it an act of gross impertinence to do so'.[74]

Concluding remarks

The use of opiate addiction as a literary device in the most familiar Victorian novels had overwhelmingly negative intentions and connotations. The addict, who might be male or female, was a tragic character portraying ruin, sickness and loss. This hopeless creature, seldom able to recover from his or her fall, acted as a metaphor personifying the wider general anxieties of pollution, parasitic degeneration, and creeping corruption. More specifically, the addict is used to embody and emphasise particular social and political ills: Dr Lydgate's struggle to reform medicine in

71 E.H. Mikhail, *Oscar Wilde: Interviews and Recollections* (1979), pp.161-2.
72 Oscar Wilde, *The Picture of Dorian Gray* (1891), pp.129, 146-8.
73 Mikhail, *Oscar Wildė*, p.162.
74 R. Ellman, *Oscar Wilde* (1987), pp.215-16.

Eliot's *Middlemarch*; Molly's seduction and consequent shameful destitution in *Silas Marner*; the neglect and culpable exploitation of *Nemo* in Dickens' *Bleak House*. Through these portrayals the authors revealed the contemporary fascination with threatening social questions and the need to decipher and explain them.[75]

Many of the fictional accounts of addiction were based on the personal experiences of the authors, some of whom were addicts themselves, some of whom knew or cared for addicts. The reading public was familiar with medicinal opium use and with the blurred line between that and addiction. And they would all have known of, if not actually read, De Quincey's *Confessions*, new editions of which were still being reviewed in 1885, sixty years after first publication, and being referred to as a 'favourite English and world classic'.[76] Whilst the addict became an increasingly familiar figure, he or she had begun to lose the romantically intriguing and picaresque persona of the early nineteenth century and by mid-century aroused either a pitiful contempt or an impotent compassion. The perceived nature of addiction was one of voluntary or involuntary personal decay, either being a cause for alarm, and its narration fed into cultural conceptualisations of decadence and degeneration present in post-Darwinist Victorian society.

75 Flint, *The Victorian Novelist*, pp.1-2.

76 *Times*, 15 May 1885, p.5, col.f.

Chapter Four

The Chinese Influence

News of foreign practices

An overwhelming sense of alienation became associated with habitual opium use over the nineteenth century, finding particular expression in the idea that it was a 'foreign practice'. Picaresque and exotic travellers' tales of opium-taking and its consequences were nothing new but were invested with a worrying authenticity when they began to appear more frequently, be they only visible in newspaper or magazine reports, or in the proselytising pamphlets of the anti-opium movement. The assorted high tales of tragedy, crime, and disaster which appeared in the popular press formed a substantial part of the mid-Victorian newspaper business and commanded a massive circulation.[1]

News is essential to human existence in that it links the individual to the world around him or her. It has been argued that the need for news is a function of human psychology and that the press must find a means to exploit this, to create a relationship with the reader's interests and experiences, with artistry, constant repetition and explanation.[2] A growing belief in the necessity for detailed knowledge allowed a sense of understanding of threatening social questions, and was imbued with the aim of instilling principles of compassion and responsibility. To this end the genre of social investigation not only reported on difficult issues but also provided the public with unfamiliar perspectives from which to view society.[3] It may also, by dint of its repetitiveness, have induced a sense of contemptuous familiarity. This form of news, in broad terms, need only purport to be factual, but its influence might nonetheless make a strong and permeating impact on an interested and fascinated audience.

Appearing merely to reveal a grim truth about addiction, press accounts also perpetrated a frightening myth. Whilst almost all Victorians might have been touched directly or indirectly by opium use, that behaviour was reduced and solidified into a stereotypical image of corruption. As early as 1829, beneath the headline 'A Celebrated Opium-Eater', the *Times* carried a curious piece on the death of Moustapha Shatyr, of Smyrna. It was reported that the Turk had died from the 'gradual effects of opium which he had acquired the habit of swallowing every day'. The dead man was treated as a sort of hybrid, a cross between a medical specimen and a celebrity. He was allegedly only forty years of age when he died but he was reported to have

1 L. Brown, *Victorian News and Newspapers* (1985), pp. 95-6.

2 Ibid.

3 Flint, *The Victorian Novelist*, p.2.

had the appearance of a very much older man: his body was emaciated and decrepit, his complexion corpse-like, and he had lost most of his teeth. This was a freakish creature, unable to 'rise from his bed without stimulating his frame with a dose of about half a dram'. Nevertheless, 'whilst under the influence of the drug, the expression on his face was particularly animated, and all his faculties seemed to be in a state of exaltation'.[4] This was an exotic and descriptive account more likely to entertain with a vicarious and xenophobic pleasure than to cause its readers to recoil in automatic horror.

Articles like this satisfied the prevalent interests in mystic exoticism, a romantic passion for the East, and an often-dark curiosity for all things foreign. The public appetite for xenophobic anxieties and morbid fears of disease and pollution were fed and perpetuated by plying such tales of apparently outlandish prodigies. The characters that peopled these accounts and coloured them with their seemingly bizarre habits became stock types in the public mind and were increasingly honed and freighted with symbolic significance. Public campaigns from the mid-nineteenth century were fuelled by such worrying images and the anti-opium societies had a particular use for them.

The popular press was not alone in perpetrating the foreign opium myth. In 1837 the *Lancet* printed a lecture from a series on medical jurisprudence being given at University College, London, which fabulously outdid the piece in the *Times* for sheer gothic drama. The lecturer, Professor A.T. Thomson, delivered an illustrative anecdote culled from an English ambassador who had apparently visited an opium-addicted 'Mahometan prince' in Persia. He lavishly described the palace as being richly decorated and spacious, ornamented with splendid and costly furniture, and the assembled crowds that inhabited it were superbly dressed. As the ambassador waited a 'lofty canopy' was carried in, 'covered with delicate silks and the richest Cashmere shawls', and upon this lay 'a human form to all appearance dead, except that its head was dangling loosely from side to side'. Two attendants carrying ornate vials of liquid then 'held up the head of the apparent corpse, and, after gently chafing the throat, and returning the tongue, which hung from a mouth relaxed and gaping, they poured some of the black liquor into the throat, and closed the jaws until it sank down the passage'. Eventually, after six or seven doses, the figure opened its eyes and closed its mouth voluntarily, swallowed a large amount of the fluid and, within an hour had regained some animation. The prince was soon able to explain to the bemused European that he was:

> an inveterate opium taker; I have, by slow degrees, fallen into this melancholy excess. Out of the diurnal twenty-four periods of time I continually pass eighteen in this reverie. Unable to move, or to speak, I am yet conscious, and the time passes away amid pleasing phantasies; nor should I ever awake from the wanderings of this state, had I not the faithful and attached servants, whose regard and religious duty impel them to watch my pulse. As soon as my heart begins to falter, and my breathing is imperceptible, except on a mirror, they immediately pour the solution of opium into my throat, and restore me as you have

4 *Times*, 27 August 1829, p.2, col.d.

> seen. Within four hours I shall have swallowed many ounces, and much time will not pass away ere I relapse into my ordinary torpor.[5]

Such fantastic accounts of the opiated living dead were forerunners of many similar articles calculated to entertain, repel, cajole and shame, and which appeared with increasing frequency from the 1860s onwards, coming to concentrate their attention on the Chinese opium smoker in particular. The Opium Wars of the mid-nineteenth century, Chinese immigration, and less specific fears of social pollution and poison thrust a new genre of reportage into the public arena: that of the experiences of those who had visited the two foreign countries of China and of 'Darkest England'. With semiotic synthesis the myth of the East End opium den entered into public consciousness and had lasting repercussions on perceptions of opium use and addiction.

Through a dissembling xenophobia came a demonisation of the foreignness of the characters portrayed, their lives and their environment. In 1868 the respectable *London Society* magazine carried an article entitled 'East London Opium Smokers' which reappeared twenty years later as 'An Opium Smoke in Tiger Bay' in a collection of the journalist James Greenwood's writings. It centred on the opium dens of Blue Gate Fields, a narrow lane that opened onto Shadwell at one end and St George's Street at the other. The Fields became infamous: the haunt of revellers and voyeurs alike. The place was commonly known as Tiger Bay on account of 'the number of ferocious she creatures in petticoats that lurk and lair there'. These 'tigresses … inveigle tipsy sailors from the many surrounding abominable dens … and drug and strip and rob and ill use them'.[6] Such dens were steeped in infamy and were said to be well patronised by sailors from the East who rushed to 'gratify their pent-up hunger for opium' as soon as they alighted at a Thames port. And not only these common customers came but others besides, including 'many distinguished members of the nobility and aristocracy … and it is rumoured even that Royalty itself has condescended to visit the opium-master in his modest retreat'. The anonymous author recorded a visit to the den, purportedly following in the footsteps of the Prince of Wales and his cohorts, to marvel at and satisfy:

> a strange yearning to make more intimate acquaintance with the miraculous drug concerning which there is so much whispering, and at the same time a superstitious dread of approaching it, such as, when it comes to the pinch, possesses the rustic believer in the efficacy of repeating a prayer backwards as a means of raising the devil.[7]

Some visitors, such as Greenwood, who recorded their sensational investigative forays there for the edification of the public, did confess to having tried opium, though some had only inhaled, and it had done nothing for them. Greenwood implied that to be affected one had obviously to be a particular and degenerate type. He had felt

5 *Lancet*, 1836-37, 2, pp.787-8.
6 Anon, 'East London Opium Smokers', *London Society* 1868, 14, pp.68-72.
7 Ibid.

unable to refuse the proffered pipe even though he was having second thoughts, for he was 'an Englishman' and the eyes of at least one of the 'sleepy barbarians' were on him. Furthermore, he nobly resolved to take his pipe sitting, and not reclining like the usual 'hideous figures' around him. He described the 'smoking-saloon' as:

> an awfully dilapidated little den … There was a bedstead in the room – a bedstead so large that there was left but a yard or so of space between it and the fire-place – a 'four-poster,' amply hung about with some kind of flimsy material, the original colour of which it is impossible to guess. But the bedding was more remarkable than the bedstead; for the bed was 'made' the wrong way – across the length of the bedstead instead of its width, with a long bolster; and it was covered, instead of a counterpane, with a huge breadth of fine Chinese matting [there were] a few gaudy prints on the walls, and the mantleshelf was crowded with ornaments, evidently of Oriental origin.[8]

The 'opium-master' was not, as Greenwood professed to expect, an individual of 'commanding aspect, richly costumed as a mandarin', but a mere travesty, a 'shabby, shambling middle-aged Chinaman' with a pigtail, Chinese boots and cap, all worn with 'vulgar' corduroy. The man's ruin of a wife was English, but this was only discernible by her speech, for her skin was 'dusky yellow, and tightly drawn at the nostrils and the cheek-bones'. And more, 'her organs of vision were fast losing their European shape, and assuming that which coincided with her adopted nature'.[9] In short, she was degenerating; she had mixed with an alien and had become an unnatural perversion of English womanhood. This was a patronising and hostile article; the opium-smokers were treated with great contempt. But readers were still informed as to where to find the dens, what the cost of smoking opium might be, and how they might prepare the drug; though the author suggested that to get a good smoke, one should visit those that were in the know rather than make an amateurish stab at it oneself.[10]

Blanchard Jerold and Gustave Doré published *London: A Pilgrimage* in 1872, a graphic record of their journeys into the dens, elaborately illustrated and described. Amid 'heart-breaking scenes of disease and helplessness' these two men had loitered with the 'lurking men' and 'flaunting hussies', witnessed the quarrelling and rollicking beneath the flickering lamps, and frequented a 'dreadful paved court' wherein lived an infamous 'Lascar opium smoker'. He lay sprawled 'upon the wreck of a four-poster bed … upon a mattress heaped with indescribable clothes'. At the foot of the bed there squatted a debased woman 'with a little brass lamp among the rags covering her, stirring the opium over the tiny flame'. It was all she could do to turn her head dreamily in their direction as they entered the hovel. The visitors, who referred to themselves as 'spies' on an alien world, agreed they could discern no trace of humanity, let alone femininity, in the woman's ruined face as her

8 J. Greenwood, 'An Opium Smoke in Tiger Bay', in *In Strange Company. Being the experiences of a roving correspondent* (1883), pp.218-19.

9 Ibid., pp.219-21.

10 Anon, 'East London Opium Smokers'.

'enormous grey dry lips lapped about the rough wood pipe and drew in the poison'. Her companion, the Lascar, appeared to them to be quite dead to the world. These creatures represented both the poisoned and the poisonous, exhibiting through the euphemistic language of the authors the transgression of virtually every known taboo. The apparently appalled voyeurs soon fled back to a civilised cleanliness, hailing a cab in the Whitechapel Road.[11] The nervous desire to experience and satisfy an ersatz thrill, to imagine such a vicious life and to indulge in the 'charming narcotic', might well allay one's anxieties if it were to offer a 'convenient picklock of the gates of paradise'.[12] Failing this one could savour it by just safely reading about it.

But how much of a reality were the opium dens and their frequenters? There had been Chinese living in the East End of London, mainly in Stepney, since the 1780s but for most of the nineteenth century this small community numbered less than 100 throughout Britain, although numbers increased from the 1860s. At the start of that decade there were about 150 Chinese in the whole country, the number increasing to nearly 700 in the following twenty years. By 1891 London was home to a total of only 582, of which 302 were China-born aliens. Numbers, then, were minuscule. But this very fact, together with differences in culture, language and dress, emphasised their visibility and alien status. Furthermore, as males outnumbered females by seven to one, they experienced additional hostility over the issue of miscegenation. The immigrants had continued to settle mainly in London, serving the Oriental population passing through the ports, with their lodging houses, laundries, shops and restaurants. As the dens existed mainly to serve these transients there were, in reality, very few of them and most were merely rooms attached to other businesses where recreational smoking took place, as if in a distorted version of a British social club. It was not until 1909 that London County Council by-laws were enacted to prohibit opium-smoking, and then only in licensed seamen's boarding houses, a limited reaction, which indicates a *laissez-faire* response to sensational reports.[13]

The anti-opium movement

Most of these accounts were the result, or a by-product, of a concerted anti-opium movement. Inspired by the Opium Wars of 1839-42 and 1856-58 the arguments and materials published by the campaign undoubtedly influenced British perceptions of the drug, its use and its consequences. The British and Indian governments demanded free trade in opium within China following the ending of the East India Company's monopoly in 1834. Whilst the company retained a monopoly on the cultivation and sale of the drug in India, its distribution in China remained in private hands, and it was thereby able to eschew responsibility for the enormous amounts entering that country. The first war was provoked by the British stand and by the Chinese Emperor's antagonism to the trade in 'this pernicious article'. It ended with the

11 Gustave Doré, and Blanchard Jerrold, *London: A Pilgrimage* (1872), pp.146-50.

12 Ibid.

13 Berridge and Edwards, *Opium*, p.195; Parssinen, *Secret Passions*, pp.53, 115-16.

Treaty of Nanking which provided for the opening of the treaty ports, British control of Chinese customs, and the continued, unabated importation of opium. In May 1840 William Gladstone declared that he was 'in dread of the judgments of God upon England for our national iniquity towards China', for he was passionately convinced of an 'overriding conscientious conviction of the hypocrisy of the government'. This was despite, or perhaps because of, Macaulay's argument against any attempt to 'exclude a drug which, if judiciously administered, was powerful in assuaging pain, and in promoting health, because it was occasionally used to excess by intemperate men'. Gladstone's fierce denunciation of 'Palmerston's Opium War' against the Chinese Empire was informed by his family's experience of opium use: his sister Helen's life was blighted, in part, by her chronic habit.[14] In 1857, during the second war, Lord Shaftesbury introduced the opium question in the House of Lords, asking for a judicial ruling on the legality of the trade. This point was finally established, and the war ended, with the Treaty of Tientsin the following year.[15] The voice of the anti-opium movement had waxed and waned throughout this time but its message, and the spectre of insidious destruction, had struck home and was to be periodically revived.

The 'Anti-Opium Society' had been formed in 1840, the 'Edinburgh Committee for the Suppression of the Indo-Chinese Opium Traffic' had appeared in 1859, but it was the 'Anglo-Oriental Society for the Suppression of the Opium Trade', formed in 1874, which had the greatest influence on public perception and political action.[16] The SSOT was largely a Quaker campaign originating in Birmingham. By relocating its headquarters to London, close to the Houses of Parliament and the India Office, by publishing *British Opium Policy and its Results to India and China* in 1876, and by appointing Lord Shaftesbury as its president in 1880, it established itself as a national movement. The organ of the SSOT was *The Friend of China*, published throughout the 1870s and 1880s. There are no circulation figures for the paper but the national press picked up many of its articles and its message was widely disseminated. Following the Treaty of Tientsin the main aim of the society was to fight for the abolition of the government monopoly on opium in India and the cessation of pressure on the Chinese government to continue importation of the expensive Indian product. In fact, by the 1880s, China was producing just as much

---

14 S.G. Checkland, *The Gladstones*, 3, pp.351-3. Helen Gladstone, prevented from marrying the man of her choice, lapsed into a 'depression and hysteria' which her physicians treated with laudanum. Sent away to Germany with a companion to mind her, she slid into chaos and then coma by swallowing 300 drops of laudanum before William could arrive to rescue the situation. Refusing to see him or to eat she was eventually brought back to England to be cared for 'in a state of coercion, so that she could obtain no stimulants, see only authorized persons, and be confined strictly to the diet prescribed'. Helen's room, where she lived out her days, could only be reached by way of her maid's, and in actions reminiscent of Coleridge's confinement, she threw messages out of her window and attempted to smuggle jewellery out, and opium in.

15 Berridge and Edwards, *Opium*, pp.173-5.

16 'Anglo-Oriental' was later omitted from the title.

home-grown opium as she was importing from India, and this downturn in the British trade, together with the growing ignominy associated with it, produced economic arguments that began to support the moral and ethical message of the campaigners.[17] The Archbishop of Canterbury, speaking at movement's greatest public moment, the famous Mansion House meeting of 21 October 1881, stated that 'the opium traffic ... is opposed alike to Christian morality and to the commercial interests of this country'.[18]

Descriptive accounts of journeys into a dangerous but exotic unknown tacitly acknowledged the curiosity, if not horror, they aroused, even in what passed as educational material for children. The *Ragged School Union Magazine*, whose precept was taken from Psalm lxxxii 'deliver the poor and needy; rid them out of the hand of the wicked', carried a short piece entitled 'In an Opium Den' in the September issue for 1868. The article recounts the experience of one Albert Woolf who, in the company of a police officer, visited an opium den in Whitechapel 'simply to look on'. The policeman appears quite familiar with the smells, the sights and the people there. This and other such dens were kept, Woolf reported, by Chinamen, and their patrons comprised 'not only Asiatics, but British sailors, and men and women who desire to find in opium that oblivion from care which alcoholic liquors cannot give'. The smokers were found in various states of 'intoxication', again lying in abandonment or 'jabbering' amongst themselves, and in their midst lay the ubiquitous old woman, the paradigm of complete corruption. Women are singled out as pariahs in this piece particularly, especially the mothers who gave opium as a 'quietener' to their offspring so that they might work or, 'what is equally common', might purposefully commit '*slow suicide* in the gin palaces of London'. The infants, with 'lack-lustre eye, the pale, yellow cheek, and the tottering limbs' were all destined for the 'premature grave ... being dug by their parents'. If one of these children survived its first few years it was to be expected that a taste for opium was 'so imbibed, that it becomes a habit in manhood', and the mothers would therefore 'suffer the penalty of their crime'. These sentiments and warnings were printed 'in the interest of the scholars of Ragged Schools' who, having already been thoroughly apprised of the evils of alcohol, were now faced with 'a vice still more deadly', one which had 'nearly ruined such men as Coleridge and De Quincey'.[19]

These works often promulgated the mixed and apparently contradictory messages of Christian ideals and imperialistic prejudices. Chastising harsh bigotry with the admission that 'a great many people despise the Chinese: they say they are untruthful, and sly, and cruel, and conceited, and very dirty', they followed up with the idea that, 'there is a good deal of truth in all this; but then we must remember that they are heathens'.[20] Fixing a necessary and beneficial warning in the minds of

---

17 Ibid.; Parssinen, *Secret Passions*, pp.89-90.

18 Berridge and Edwards, *Opium*, p.181.

19 Anon., *The Ragged School Union Magazine* September 1868, 20, pp.198-200.

20 Ibid., p.4.

the impressionable also often entailed fixing rigid, unforgiving and persistent ideas about others:

> Although opium is a poison, it is very useful in medicine; it soothes the most violent pain, and gives sleep when nothing else can. But what would you think of a man who took medicine when he was quite well, and tried to send himself to sleep in the day-time, when he ought to be doing his work? You would call him a very foolish man. But this is just what many people do. They eat or smoke opium, and it makes them feel very comfortable at first, and gives them the most delightful dreams. But when they wake up they feel very wretched, and if they keep on taking it for a long time, it makes them quite ill, and at last kills them. Confirmed opium-smokers walk about with bent figures, and pinched, yellow faces, and become in time quite unable to do their daily work. Opium is very expensive, and using so much of it makes them poor; and yet they feel they must have more of it to stop the horrible pains which the poison itself has given them. When they have no more money to buy it, they steal it, or steal something else to sell in exchange for it, for the love of opium deadens a man's conscience and makes him ready to do any wicked deed ... smokers have been known to sell their wives or little children so as to buy opium. When a man begins to smoke it, he thinks he will be able to take only a little; but after a time he finds that opium has become his master, and he its slave, and then it is too late to stop.[21]

Children were asked to remember that the British had 'no right to force the Chinese to take anything – even a good thing – *against their will*', and 'no right to *poison* the Chinese, even if they asked us to poison them'.[22] And they were encouraged to do more than just absorb these frightening stories for their own future benefit: they could play an active part in suppressing the evil by selling anti-opium tracts; telling others about the evident dangers; and by praying for the practice and the trade in opium to China to stop. 'Do not think', wrote another anonymous author of one of these pamphlets, 'that you are too young to help. I know a little boy, only six years old, who has been interested in opium for more than a year'.[23] No missionary was considered too young or insignificant and none, of course, too grand: the Bishop of Durham was one of the earliest supporters of the campaign, and the Archbishop of Canterbury played a prominent role.[24]

There was, and is now, an analogy to be drawn between the slavery of addiction to opium and the slavery of a people to despotic government. The Lord Mayor of London, closing the Mansion House meeting of 1881, predicted that, 'in the course of a little time we shall see in relation to the opium traffic what we have seen with regard to slavery – that it will be put down'.[25] An anonymous Chinese, resident in London and writing for the *Times* and the *Friend of China* in 1875, had remarked that 'people living in a free country like England are apt to forget' how others might be subject to a 'despotic monarchical Government without the consent, and even

21 Ibid., p.6.
22 Ibid., p.13.
23 Anon., *Poppies: A talk with English boys and girls about opium* (1860), p.13.
24 Berridge and Edwards, *Opium*, p.179.
25 H. Sultzberger, ed., *All About Opium* (1884), p.20.

against the expressed wishes of the people'. Many of his countrymen were subject to the insidious but tenacious nature of opium addiction and deserved the understanding and sympathy of the British, whom he considered 'guilty of national complicity in this pernicious [opium] trade'.[26] Summoning up the English conceit of a 'love of right and justice' he professed himself unable to believe them capable of being 'perfectly aware of the evils and miseries caused to China by the use of opium'. Yet still they persisted in extracting a 'revenue of six millions sterling annually' from this exploitation of his countrymen and women who demonstrated their humanity by 'being frail and prone to evil'.[27] It was no coincidence that the campaign style of the S.S.O.T. conformed closely to the model established by the Anti-Slavery Society: that of a pressure group cultivating both public antagonism towards the opium trade and aiming for direct political action through parliamentary entreaty.[28]

The experiences of another English slave to opium who had begun his habit in China were dissected in *The Friend of China*, and the unfortunate man's 'fall' was said to have robbed him of a 'good position in life' and of his 'excellent abilities'. This article, 'An essay on the Consequences to be expected from the opium trade as carried on between England, India, and China', was allegedly written by a Chinese and published in 1876. It was intended to engage the moral sensibilities and anxieties of the reader by exposing the many dangers of addiction and by suggesting the possibility that the condition could spread, like a noxious contagion, if, 'at some future date such men ... lead others to smoke opium'.[29] But the main objective of the piece was to attack and condemn the British commercial exploitation of the opium trade. The economic and moral arguments were impossible to disentangle: they soaked the trade in shameful odium and preserved in the public mind the nascent, stereotypical image of the ruined drug addict.

As the fortunes of the anti-opium campaign waxed and waned its influence remained, whilst, conversely, there existed no concerted, propagandising pro-opium movement in opposition. Even so, letters from interested individuals appeared in the press, such as the following in the *Pall Mall Gazette* on 13 November 1879, which objected to the climate of fear and loathing:

> The denouncers of the drug are apt to get under the influence of a fixed idea, or, to speak in vulgar parlance, "they get opium on the brain", and whenever they see a person unwell who happens to be an opium smoker they at once attribute his illness to his habit of smoking opium - "Post hoc, ergo propter hoc". On the other hand, it is equally incontrovertible that thousands of hardworking people are indebted to opium smoking for the continuance of lives agreeable to themselves and useful to society.

---

26 'What The Chinese Think About Opium', *The Friend of China*, October 1875, pp.195, 197.

27 Ibid., pp.199, 200.

28 Berridge and Edwards, *Opium*, p.179.

29 *The Friend of China*, April 1876, 12, p.340.

Henry Sultzberger, a foreign commission merchant who dealt in commercial opium as well as many other commodities, had observed what he called the 'ever-increasing attacks made by the well-known Anti-Opium Society on this most unjustly abused article' and decided to redress the balance. In 1884, at his own expense, he published *All About Opium*, a small volume of collected articles and letters, ostensibly designed to allow 'everyone to judge for himself on its merits' but with obvious pro-opium leanings. Sultzberger saw opium traffic as the victim, the 'undefended prisoner … looked upon as simply foredoomed', its advocates lacking 'that systematic cohesion … which gives so much apparent importance' to its detractors. His arguments included what he considered to be the laws of supply and demand, the effects of high duties which encouraged smuggling, and, speciously, the impossibility of '*forcing*' opium on the Chinese '*in particular*'. They had, as a people, a long history of opium use and a government that 'sought to prohibit it only so soon as they saw that their silver was rapidly leaving the country'.[30] Thus he disingenuously shifted any ethical responsibility from his own shoulders and those of his fellow merchants and supporters of the trade.

The problem of addiction inherent in the opium trade was sidestepped and the use of the drug reduced to 'merely a question of geography and race, and not of morality in the least'.[31] In a letter to the *Times* in 1881, reprinted in Sultzberger's volume, Sir George Birdwood, a former medical student in Edinburgh, claimed it for a fact that humanity had a 'universal craving … for some kind of stimulant' and if 'we are always being called upon to appreciate the divine bounty … of cereal and pulse grains' then, surely, 'narcotic stimulants, which are to be found in almost every natural order of plants' must be recognised as *designed* to 'make glad the heart of man'. He was not, he protested, approving the use of narcotics, but dismissing their 'falsely imputed immorality'. Taking opium was, he argued, 'absolutely harmless … a perfectly innocuous indulgence', and, though he had known cases of 'desperate suffering, resulting, apparently from excess … these cases were always of moral imbeciles … addicted to other forms of depravity [and] inherently enervated.' Instances of 'evil' consequent on opium use were extremely rare he thought, and, in his opinion, were not to be found amongst 'sound, hale people, in comfortable circumstances' who, though they indulged, led healthy lives and never suffered from habitual use. Any *habitué* was, therefore, the architect of his or her own demise and was most probably destined, by virtue of inherited blood, to suffer and fall.

This adulterated mix of medical and religious assumption often found support within that marginal part of the medical profession that had come to specialise in addiction. George Beard MD, in his works in the 1870s and 1880s on nervous exhaustion and on the effects of stimulants and narcotics, claimed that he was also making a 'contribution to sociology', promoting discussion of heredity, race, education, religion, legislation, morals and social customs. The effects of drugs were, according to Beard, 'modified by race [and] temperament', so that in the East, where

30 Sultzberger, *All About Opium*, pp.vii, 101.

31 Sir George Birdwood's letter to the *Times*, 26 December 1881, ibid., p.25.

opium was produced and 'habitually used among about 400,000,000 inhabitants', it appeared to him 'to do much less evil than with us. The masses would appear to be injured by it far less than would be supposed'. In the West 'few indeed' could use opium 'for a long time without harm', and the results carried some of the most 'deplorable consequences' because it 'expends greater force' in civilised nations than in 'barbarism'.[32]

Even at the very end of the century, despite Beard's assurances of calm and rational discussion by 'well-trained minds' on the subject of opium use, Oscar Wilde's accounts of opium-smoking in *The Picture of Dorian Gray* (1890), and in his play *For the Love of the King a Burmese Masque* (1892), remained imbued with expected ingredients of alien fantastry which perpetrated the myth of the exotic yet repulsive Oriental opium-smoker:

> At the home of the Chinese Wizard, Hip Loong, by the river – a place filled with Chinese things: Dragons of gold with eyes of jade ... Buddhas of gigantic size ... swinging banners with fringes of many-coloured stones, lanterns with glass sides on which are painted grotesque figures. The air is full of the scent of joss-sticks. The wizard reclines on a divan, inhaling opium slowly, clothed with the subdued gorgeousness of China ... He has the appearance of a pickled walnut. His forehead is a lattice-work of wrinkles. His pigtail, braided with red, is twisted round his head. His hands are as claws. The effect is weird, unearthly.[33]

And these by now familiar, parodic and caricatured stereotypes continued to be fed to the public through magazines, newspapers and religio-political pamphlets. In the 1890s the first volume of *The Strand Magazine* carried a salacious account of 'A Night in an Opium Den', written by the anonymous author of such works as 'A Dead Man's Diary'. 'Yes', began the daringly triumphant adventurer, 'I have smoked opium'. And, what is more, attempting to claim investigative verisimilitude, he maintained that the deed took place in the very same den visited by Charles Dickens, and that he had used the very same pipe 'which had the honour of making that distinguished novelist sick'.[34] The Chinese proprietor of the den was purported to have an 'evil look': he had 'parchment-coloured features ... small and cunning eyes [that] twist and turn so horribly' and a fixed, 'bland and penetrating smile ... which threatened to distort permanently his features'. The ubiquitous ill-lit, 'reeking hole' with mattresses and opium paraphernalia made their appearances and, as an added horrifying touch, there blasphemously hung a 'coarsely-coloured and hideous print of the crucifixion'. The 'yellow' and stupefied Chinese and Malays sprawled about the room, the proprietor meticulously prepared the pipes, and a 'young and by no

32 G. Beard, *Stimulants and Narcotics; Medically, Physically, and Morally Considered* (1871), pp.1, 38, 57; *A Practical Treatise on Nervous Exhaustion (Neurasthenia): Its Symptoms, Nature, Sequences, Treatment* (1880), pp.xiv, 120.

33 Wilde, *For the Love of the King a Burmese Masque* (1892), Act III, Scene II, pp.27-8.

34 Anon., 'A Night in an Opium Den', *The Strand Magazine*, 1891, 1, pp.624-7.

means ill-looking Englishwoman' was soon present. She, with little or no modesty according to the reporter, began, quite immodestly, to 'tickle' the filthy smokers, provoking 'unearthly, and uncontrollable laughter'. Diverting her attention to the reporter she took mental stock of his appearance and wealth and he recounted that, when he woke from his stupor later that evening, he discovered she had divested him of his boots, hat and umbrella. But it was in the description of his opium dreams that his pastiche was revealed: he recalled, he wrote, a 'sensation of floating, as on a cloud … of seeing, through vistas of purple and gold … the fabled "Blessed Isles", stretching league beyond league afar … and a vision of white warm arms and wooing bosoms'. De Quincey, whom the author conjures up for credibility alongside Dickens, would have thrown up his white warm arms in dismay at this crass representation.

Medicine and the Chinese influence

The medical profession made its own forceful contribution to the anti-opium campaigns and to the formation of the opium myth and its stereotypes. From the 1840s onwards various medical journals were carrying accounts of, and opinions on, opium-smoking, opinions which were undoubtedly intended to widen and inform both the medical and the political debates. In February 1842, as the first opium was coming to an end, a Dr Johnson delivered a paper, 'On Opium-Smoking among the Chinese', to the Westminster Medical Society. It was written by a G. H. Smith, a surgeon in Penang, and abstracts of it were subsequently printed in the *Lancet* and the *Medico-Chirurgical Review and Journal*.[35] The practice was introduced as a 'destructive vice' almost utterly impossible to relinquish if the 'dreadful habit' had taken hold. Once acquired, it affected more than the individual, opening up an 'immense source of revenue to the East India Company', and contributing to the 'immense and incalculable' quantity of opium smuggled.

Smith recorded faithfully the processes involved in preparing the drug, the methods of smoking, and the amounts of opium consumed, but he used the florid language and astonished tone of the European traveller to describe the people who smoked, their reasons for smoking and the consequences of their habit. Laying the blame for the practice amongst the Chinese on their 'remarkably social and luxurious disposition', he believed many fell prey to it out of mere politeness. He claimed that parents indulged their children in an effort to 'prevent them from running into other vices still more detestable … to which the Chinese are more prone than, perhaps, any people on earth'. Thus he painted them as victims, but as ignorant and vicious barbarians too, a most definite race apart.

With the triteness of accumulated, mixed, and well-worn assumptions he suggested that young Chinese men smoked opium because they believed it 'heightens and prolongs venereal pleasures', whilst older men used it to drown their

35 *Lancet*, 1841-42, 1, pp.707-10; *Medico-Chirurgical Review and* Journal, 1842, 36, pp.583-7.

cares and troubles, 'in an indescribably pleasurable feeling of indifference to all around'. Women rarely indulged and if they did they were, naturally, 'abandoned prostitutes' and their offspring 'weak, stunted, and decrepit'. The rich smoked in special, elegant saloons, whilst the poor went to 'gloomy abodes of vice and misery ... most intolerable to the olfactories' of the more refined and civilised European races. Smith's descriptions of these places were remarkably similar to the journalistic pictures painted of the dens in Bluegate Fields, London. The smokers displayed 'stupor, forgetfulness, general deterioration of all the mental faculties, emaciation, debility, sallow complexion, lividity of lips and eyelids, languor and lack-lustre of eye [their] appetite either destroyed or depraved'.[36]

This pathologically paranoiac image of the alien Oriental and his devastating habits had great imaginative persistence, and opium's 'pernicious effect on the constitution ... of its victims' was too great to dismiss. Even a 'strong and healthy' Chinese soon became 'little better than an idiot skeleton', and the 'pain they suffer when deprived of the drug after long habit, no language can explain'.[37] These opinions were constantly repeated, despite the knowledge that De Quincey's eulogy of the drug had proved that the reality could be different, and that English opium-taking was no different.[38]

Dr Johnson's notes, which accompanied this paper, provoked a professional discussion at the Westminster Medical Society but made no comment on the negative portrayal of the Chinese. It was widely and traditionally accepted that differences in race, climate, diet, and culture affected physiological responses to drugs, and the questions of race and of the '*habitual abuse*' of opium, never mind how graphically and repugnantly they were described, were dismissively glossed over and accepted as a given. The apparently curious practice of opium-smoking, 'little known in this country', and how it might prove more medicinally effective than taking the drug by mouth, were the questions that provoked professional interest. The argument focused solely on the premise that, if smoking proved more medicinally and immediately effective than taking the drug into the stomach, then that was 'no reason against its occasional exhibition as a remedial agent'.[39] The *Lancet* carried articles in 1839 and 1842 suggesting this method, despite its known 'various evils' and the warning that 'so fascinating is the influence of this noxious drug, that many would prefer death to exclusion from smoking it'.[40] The experience of opium addiction remained a controversial and obscure curiosity whilst the medical profession sought, on the whole, to confine itself to questions of therapeutic technique.

The argument for inhalation was proposed again thirty years later, albeit anonymously, in a short pamphlet, *What opium feels like. By one who has tried it*

36 Ibid.

37 *Bell's Pharmaceutical Journal*, 1848, 7, p.292.

38 N. Leask, *British Romantic Writers and the East: Anxieties of Empire* (1993), p.171.

39 *Lancet*, 1841-42, 1, p.710.

40 Ibid., 1839-40, 1, p.418; 1842-3, 2, p.113.

(1870). The author suggested that 'it might be useful if the subject were investigated by medical men, to see if opium smoking might not be found a convenient way of administering the drug to patients who otherwise cannot take it without the stomach being upset'. A medical-supplier, Farmers & Rogers of Regent St, was even offering, during the 1860s, an opium pipe with 'all appurtenances, including lamp, vessel for oil, boxes for opium, etc.', for ten shillings and sixpence. As late as the 1890s Benjamin Ward Richardson conducted a survey of the various means of taking the drug but, on visiting the dens of East London, chose, for moral and political reasons, to condemn the practice of opium-smoking.[41] This was a serious discussion, often forcibly argued, and opium-taking continued to be alternately promoted and decried throughout the second half of the nineteenth century. Nonetheless it was almost always accompanied by the extra weight of xenophobic ballast, as though the subject could no longer be approached without a protective patina of moral anxiety.

Other contemporary observers, however, disagreed with what they saw as a cavalier treatment of the potential problem of addiction. A surgeon, writing to the *Lancet* with an extract from the private journal of his travels in China in the 1880s, made it emphatically plain that 'the habitual use of opium ... cannot fail to produce the most injurious effects upon the constitution'. Using now familiar images and language, he expressed the professional opinion that 'the peculiar languid and vacant expression, the sallow and shrivelled countenance ... the general emaciated and withered appearance of the body, easily distinguish the confirmed opium-smoker'.[42] Another British physician, practicing in China, considered the 'habitual use of opium ... most disastrous, alike in its physical and moral results'. He reported that he had received hundreds of requests for help from addicts wanting 'deliverance from the habit'.[43] The *British Medical Journal* carried a piece on an English gentleman aged fifty-three, and addicted for thirty-five years, who had acquired the habit on visiting China at the age of thirteen. He had 'discovered by experiment the fascination of the drug ... and commenced the habit as a luxury'. In later life, when serving as an officer in the British army in India, his daily dose had allegedly risen to at least two hundred grains a day.[44] Yet another physician declared that all opium-smokers seemed to him to be ashamed of their habit and he was asked 'over and over again if [he] could cure the craving'.[45] A Chinese commentator with a large number of habituated friends and relatives, whilst believing that the condition was not 'insuperable' if a victim could be compelled to break it or 'had sufficient determined resolution', denied that even moderate use was without its ill effects.[46] It was argued that addiction was not only a Chinese weakness but that it might also infect a respectable European, and the presence of the East London opium dens seemed to support this.

41 Berridge and Edwards, *Opium*, pp.196, 198, 204.
42 *Lancet*, 1881-82, 1, pp.820-2.
43 *British Medical Journal*, 2 July 1881, p.30.
44 Ibid., October 1881, p.716.
45 *Blackwood's Edinburgh Magazine*, April 1896, p.571.
46 *The Friend of China*, October 1875, pp.193, 199.

Concluding remarks

The portraits of opium dens and opium addicts that appeared in novels, newspaper articles, magazines and journals presented the reader with the same lost figures, the same sulphurous yellow and wizened visages of smokers and the same poisonous, sickly atmospheres. The corruption, filth, degeneration, and the revulsion felt by the visitor from some cleaner, purer, rational, Christian English place, all made their rhetorical appearances time and time again. Ideas of foreignness and sickness were wedded together by these descriptive devices and they acted directly on xenophobic and nosophobic anxieties. The repeated use of these images succeeded in fixing a trite idea of repugnant degradation in the mind of the public, but they also allowed a contemptuous familiarity to distance the misery and prevent understanding and empathy. A reality had informed the imaginary and a generic literary form had arisen.

Such burlesque portrayals excited the fears and dangers of a social cacotopia. The very passivity of opium-smoking had become a positive threat, and the perceived rise of the practice in England, fuelled by xenophobic accounts, was understood to be a symptom of racial degeneration. Even the persistent use of the word 'yellow' to describe the Chinese coincided with the colour of decadence. The figures of the 'weak and unmanly' English smoker, whose 'depraved appetite' was satiated in the quasi-mythical East London opium den, and the deviant and corrupted femininity of his female counterpart were paraded before the anxious imagination of the reading public. These stereotypes had become a powerful propaganda tool for the S.S.O.T. and clarified a composite image of the opium-smoker. The public was offered a fixed and definite type together with particular characteristics and behaviours that would remain associated with the drug addict. The mix of moral concern and fearful disgust was overlaid with the politics and economics of imperialism. At the very end of the nineteenth century came a comment on the availability of opium that still reverberates today: 'in their failure to legalise the trade, all parties conspired to foster its attendant evils. That is abundantly clear to us now.'[47]

47 'The English in China' in *Blackwood's Magazine*, January 1901, p.68.

PART II
The Medical History of Addiction in Nineteenth-Century Britain

Chapter Five

Poisonous Drugs and the Medical Profession in the Nineteenth Century

They love not poison that do poison need
Shakespeare, King Richard II, Act 5, Scene 6

The poisonous beginnings of 'use and abuse'

From the early nineteenth century there was a constant and increasingly urgent search for a greater understanding of properties and effects of opium. Case-histories of accidental and intentional opium poisonings, articles on toxicology, and reports of clinical lectures, began to litter the pages of the growing number of medical journals and the popular press. These accounts emerged from an abiding tradition of discussing the properties and effects of opium, were often fraught with controversy, and formed part of the vanguard of the mid-nineteenth-century shift in the understanding of addiction. The debate was both an expression of the nascent struggle for monopoly between the different branches of the medical profession and a portent of medical anxieties to come.

During the early nineteenth century, with the process of medical professionalisation and the publication of new medical journals, the debate over the drug was beginning to enter a larger, more critically concerned professional and public consciousness which would begin to crystallize in theories, treatments and attitudes from the mid-nineteenth century onwards. The 'so-called' age of medical reform, recognised as a period stretching from the late seventeenth to the twentieth century, encompassed this process and was unrelenting and often vitriolic, rich in accusation and counter-accusation.[1] Before the Apothecaries Act of 1815 and the medical registration measures of 1858 there were no precise parameters to the term 'qualified medical practitioner', and the struggle for status inevitably included the designation and categorisation of the sick and of disease in order to legitimise the orthodox physician's claims. The controversy over the newly defined disease of addiction, particularly from the mid-nineteenth century onwards, and attempts to control and regulate opiate use, were part of this process and were reflected in the medical journals and popular press of the time.

1 I. Loudon, 'The vile race of quacks with which this country is infected', in W.F. Bynum and R. Porter, eds, *Medical Fringe and Medical Orthodoxy* (1987), pp.106-28.

The disease entity of addiction emerged from the medical identification and elaboration of perceived dangers that were social, political, and economic, as well as physiological and psychological. Notions of drug abuse and addiction were enveloped early on in scientific and moral uncertainty, in debate that resisted clarification, persisting into the second half of the nineteenth century and beyond. But whereas later work focused on the concept of addiction and its treatment, its emergence is to be found in earlier works on poisoning and its remedies. Increasing awareness and anxieties over actual and perceived poisons and their effects charged the popular and scientific imaginations and heightened the desire to inform and control. Opium addiction was one aspect of this cultural and medical trend, and it was a pivotal aspect, a link between experience and science.

Medical knowledge was not an autonomous system of thought: social, cultural, political and commercial spheres influenced the direction and choice of physicians in diseases and therapies.[2] As the medical profession sought to validate itself and expand it gave rise to medical specialisms, one of which was toxicology, a discipline that illustrated one of the ways in which nineteenth-century medical development was associated with concepts of public health and safety. The infamous court case in 1832 which detailed the opium habit of the Earl of Mar gave toxicology and addiction a greater public profile and ensured that these subjects were not treated in a purely scientific manner, despite attempts by many medical commentators to confine them to that sphere.

Responses to accidental poisonings, deliberate poisonings, and suicides made the task of empirical understanding harder still. The properties and effects of opium were known to produce some often disturbing symptoms in users, and provoked an array of responses to its known benefits and disadvantages. The qualities it possessed were, according to the physicians themselves, imperfectly understood and difficult to quantify scientifically. Primarily concerned with the physiological effects of opium, they could not help but lace their opinions with moral warnings and anxieties as to the consequences of incautious and 'illicit' use.

Early warnings

A strident warning about the 'general and shameful abuse of opium' appeared in a '*Report from the General Hospital near Nottingham*', published in the *Edinburgh Medical and Surgical Journal* in 1808.[3] This was one of the earliest concerned and public diatribes in a debate on unorthodox drug use that began with medical anxieties over imperfect knowledge and control of certain substances. It continues today and many of the early impressions and arguments are revisited in cyclical fashion, albeit using different language.

2 A. Wear, 'Making sense of health and the environment in early modern England', in A. Wear, ed., *Medicine in Society* (1992), pp.119-47.

3 *Edinburgh Medical and Surgical Journal*, 1808, 4, pp.271-2.

The anonymous physician wrote fervently about the effects of unrestricted opium-taking, discussing his findings with restrained anger and anxiety. This was 'abuse' on the part of, in particular, the 'poorer class' of people, and was distinctly different in his opinion, from the respectable, regulated and knowledgeable orthodox system of treatment by a medical practitioner. The consequences for adults who abused opium and 'habituated themselves to it', and the infant mortality that he also ascribed to it, exercised him sorely and he believed that 'very few are sensible to what an extent this practice prevails in large manufacturing towns'. Opium was a remedy in the trained hands of physicians but a 'deadly poison' in the grasp of the common people; the druggist's shop was the 'grand emporium' for the careless sale of the drug. The culpable druggist might spend nearly half his time employed in forming and dispensing opium compounds, a 'great incentive to indolence', to the unwary or feckless. In his desire to warn his readers of the dangers, the physician assured them that these drugs always 'finally bring [their] votaries to poverty and disease', and provided them with an alarming though rough estimate of the quantities sold to the 'poorer class', one that ran to 'upwards of 200lb. of opium, and above 600 pts. of Godfrey's cordial ... in the year'. The prevailing high cost of the drug, he thought, might have had some limiting effect on the numbers of accidental poisonings of infants, but it was small restraint on the adults who would 'pawn their clothes that they may be enabled to purchase this delectable charm, this momentary balm to all cares and disappointments, which obtunds the faculties and undermines the sentient principle'.[4]

In October 1816 Dr Marshall Hall published his article 'Contributions to Diagnosis', offering his 'practical observations' on, among other things, *The Effects of the Habit of giving Opiates on the Infantine Constitution.*[5] He freely admitted that his observations were, however, sometimes 'rather desultory, and of a mixed nature', and it is clear that his use of language was distinctly less scientific and more emotively and romantically florid than later, similar works were to be. Hall described, for example, a six-month-old infant whose mother had begun what he termed the 'pernicious practice' of giving it an anodyne every night to promote sleep, so reducing her child to 'a shocking disfigured appearance'. The child's 'whole face', he wrote, 'is at once aged, haggard, and painful to see [and there] is an entire want of that appearance of intelligence observed in infants in general even of this age'. He recorded the death of a second infant from this 'baneful practice', a tiny unfortunate whose skin was shrivelled and who was the 'most remarkable living miniature of old age, in the female countenance, that can be imagined'. The babies were prescribed a remedial regimen, being 'made to abstain from [their] anodyne, and to take small doses of calomel and of magnesia daily, with a nutritious diet'. It is evident that the physician was truly disturbed by the dangers of drugging unhappy infants and he clearly intended his readers to be equally horrified. In the knowledge

4 Ibid.

5 *Edinburgh Medical and Surgical Journal*, 1816, 12, p.423.

that his treatments were inadequate he used his article to draw attention to the misery he had encountered as his best weapon against the practice.

The rousing language and detail used in these articles did much to alert the reader to a hidden potential danger and to an underworld of neglect and despair that seemed to call out for investigation and regulation.[6] But it loses its force for present-day readers when we become aware that the writer had a very different conception of classes of poisons to that provided for the modern observer. There was little or no recognition of any escalation of degrees of potency and harm in different drugs; rather, each drug was deemed to possess particular 'special powers' which might affect its victim idiosyncratically according to 'different temperaments [which] appear in a certain degree to influence the performance of various actions differing in their nature'.[7]

In this notion of the reaction of the individual we can clearly see the thread of the medical theory of humouralism, based on the classical authority of Galen, which had been in decline since the mid-eighteenth century and was being replaced by chemical and mechanical explanations of the body. Humouralism was of the Aristotelian world, a qualitative system based on four causes: the material, formal, efficient and final causes. Composed of four qualities, hot, cold, dry, and moist, in combination they produced the elements, water (moist and cold), earth (dry and cold), air (moist and hot), and fire (hot and dry). The humours were phlegm (moist and old), blood (moist and hot), yellow bile (hot and dry), black bile (dry and cold). Ill health would result when the humours were imbalanced and out of harmony.

Under this principle of humoural individualism, which held that everyone possessed their own peculiar and innate crasis, it was acknowledged that one drug or remedy might suit some but harm others.[8] Present-day drug theories concur. It was understood that any individual who took opium, 'suffer[ing] it to remain for a period that, in many persons would prove fatal', and who subsequently recovered, had this 'invariably attributed by the patient's friends and medical attendant to the individual's constitution in opposition to any known physiological principles'.[9] Hence the author of the 1808 Nottingham report could suggest that to those who were addicted to opium it 'becomes, like tea, or the pipe'. Even if there existed those who 'esteem *tea* very salutary, by giving "a temporary excitement, an intellectual and cloudless inebriety" ... and assert that many lovers of this beverage have lived to a good old age', these arguments, he maintained, were not to be considered proof of benignity. Furthermore, the apparently salutary effects of tea could, for some unfortunate individuals, 'with equal propriety, be applied to vinous or spiritous potations ... and

6 There were no restrictions on opium use until the first Pharmacy Act was passed in 1868.

7 'On the Utility of a Knowledge of the Temperaments in Connection with the Diagnosis and Treatment of Disease', *Lancet*, 1846, 1, pp.360-1.

8 B. Harrison, *Drink and the Victorians: The Temperance Question in England 1815-1872* (1994), p.298.

9 Ibid.

even to opium itself'.[10] Whilst it was already being argued, therefore, that it was not the particular drug which could cause harm but the individual temperament and predisposition to addiction, the control of poisons was also paramount to the medical profession and its consolidation.

Graduates of the Edinburgh Medical School were prominent in this new field and many of them had studied in Paris under the pioneering physicians Magendie and Orfila. Orfila's *Traité des Poisons* was reviewed in 1817 in the *Edinburgh Medical and Surgical Journal*, and English translations of Magendie's *Formulary for the Preparation and Employment of New Remedies* were appearing in the late 1820s. These works were purportedly based on experience and experimentation, adopting increasingly scientific methodologies in their approach. Despite this they attracted critical attention, and in a review of Orfila's work it was suggested that the doctor entertained 'somewhat peculiar' opinions on the properties of opium. He had posited the idea that the drug, 'in a large dose, ought not to be considered either as a narcotic or as a stimulant poison', but that it exercised 'a particular mode of action for which [there is] no name'. In arguing that in some cases, 'depending on idiosyncrasy', the effects of opium were unpredictable, Orfila seemed to be in agreement with the Nottingham doctor who had penned the local hospital report in 1808.

The case of the Earl of Mar

The scandalous court case in 1832 that revealed the thirty-year opium addiction of the Earl of Mar gave the emerging specialism of toxicology a very public platform. This infamous case made opium addiction a subject of intense interest for medico-legal, social, and political reasons, and revealed issues of shame and secrecy, morality and health. It also exposed the paucity of medical knowledge of opium and motivated the profession to intensify its experimental and observational investigations into the drug and its properties and effects.

On 9 March 1832 the banking establishment of Sir William Forbes and Company raised an action against the Edinburgh Life Assurance Company for refusing to honour a bill of insurance totalling £7000, drawn on John Thomas Erskine, 14th Earl of Mar, on 26 September 1826.[11] The policy was held by the bankers as security for a loan issued to the Earl, who died of jaundice and dropsy two years later, aged fifty-seven, in September 1828.[12] Following his death the late Earl's insurances

10 *Edinburgh Medical and Surgical Journal*, 1808, 4, pp.271-2.

11 Bell and Bradsute, *Cases Decided in the Court of Session*, 12 November 1831 - 12 July 1832, x, pp. 451-65.

12 In the relevant court papers, SRO reference CS248/3048, there are about 130 parties listed as claimants on the estate, either as creditors or trustees. Litigation in the cases brought by the Earl's claimants extended over at least sixty years with interlocutors being pronounced as late as 2 March 1889, including a decree on the claim by the late Earl's daughter, the Right Honourable Lady Frances Jemima Erskine or Goodeve, against the Right Honourable John Francis Miller, 15th Earl of Mar.

were claimed by his creditors, but the Edinburgh Life Assurance Company received information about their client's long-standing habit of using laudanum 'to excess', and that he had been so indulging at the time he effected his policy. The records of the Court of Sessions detail the directions put by the Judge to the jury, being, first, 'whether a question regarding habits remained unanswered', secondly, whether the life insured was 'more than usually hazardous', and, thirdly, whether the fact that a possibly 'dangerous habit of opium-eating ... not disclosed' would render any insurance policy invalid.[13] The Edinburgh Life Assurance Company eventually lost the case on a technicality, being found liable due to their having departed from the usual practice and precaution of insurance companies when requesting information on a client's general 'habits'. The trial had 'involved no question of law, but was to be decided by the rules of common sense', and these rested on the medical evidence given in respect of the possible effects of a long-standing habit of opium-eating.[14]

Professor Robert Christison of Edinburgh, toxicologist and author of a *Treatise on Poisons* (1829), was one of several medical practitioners applied to by the parties concerned for information and opinions at the trial. His account of the proceedings appeared in a series of lectures on 'Medical Jurisprudence' in the *Edinburgh Medical and Surgical Journal* in 1832, adding considerably to the growing debate on the use of opium, and bringing into the public gaze the spectre of chronic unorthodox consumption.[15] Christison set the tone of his article with the uncompromising statement that he found it a 'singular' matter how 'very little is known by the medical profession of the effects of the practice of eating opium or drinking laudanum on health or longevity'. He lamented the fact that the information supplied by the physicians and put forward at the trial consisted of little more than presumptive statements and matters of opinion. To compound matters it appeared that 'no one had any direct experience on the subject', or, if they had, they were not prepared to disclose it in a public arena. The trial exposed the secrecy and shame already associated with addiction, and the yawning chasm in the field of medico-legal toxicology.

Christison used De Quincey's confessional experiences of opium addiction as a case-history, remarking that although he thought it a 'very poetical' work, he also believed it to be a unique and 'faithful picture of the phenomena'.[16] Christison affirmed, however, that physicians employed the drug 'differently' and not 'idiosyncratically' in the pursuit of 'material excitement', and thus emphasised a distinction between scientific use and personal indulgence, but without casting any serious aspersions on the latter. With such information and preconceptions as were available to him, he arrived at his conclusions through a form of medical common sense. He could not,

13 Bell and Bradsute, pp.451-2.

14 Christison, Professor of Medical Jurisprudence and Police in the University of Edinburgh, 'Article X, Cases and Observations in Medical Jurisprudence - Case X. On the effects of Opium-eating on Health and Longevity', *Edinburgh Medical and Surgical Journal*, 1832, 37, p.124.

15 Ibid., pp.123-35

16 Christison, 'Of the Action of Opium and the Symptoms it Excites in Man', in *A Treatise on Poisons* (1829), pp.645-63.

he wrote, bring himself to agree that the habitual use of a drug with such apparently poisonous effects as opium, should be left to those who 'use it habitually' and who live in 'so miserable a state during the intervals of using it'.[17] Though he understood opium-eating with the physician's mentality of 'Body and Gut', and not with the mentality of the opium addict, he could still admit that his profession possessed 'little or no precise information on the matter'.[18]

Despite the apparent lack of *a priori* knowledge, Christison maintained that the practice of opium-eating did in fact prevail to a 'very considerable extent both among the lower orders and better ranks of society'. The reasons put forward for this were that the poor combined the habit with excessive drinking, thereby rendering accurate observation almost impossible, whilst their masters in general concealed it 'sedulously' from their medical attendants.[19] The Earl of Mar, a solitary, shrewd and studious man had, 'with a little pains', found it quite easy to 'conceal for years [his] confirmed habit of opium-eating, with all its consequences', from his friends, medical attendants and staff. He saw so little company that, 'from first to last', none of his associates could give any account of his habits, bar a Mr Miller who occasionally dined with him, and he remarked only that the Earl drank no more than other men. The only physician to have attended the Earl in the two years before his death stated that his health had 'from one cause or another, long been in an infirm state' and that his constitution appeared to be broken down but 'without any specific disease being present'. The Earl's gardener, coal-manager, gamekeeper and woodman all declared that the Earl was often out on his estates, superintending and sometimes assisting them in their work for an hour or two every afternoon, yet not one of them had noticed any 'stupor or operation of narcotic drugs' (suggesting that people from all walks of life were familiar with and could readily recognise such symptoms). But, from the evidence of the person who had been closest to him, it emerged that the Earl had been 'much addicted to this habit' for almost all his adult life. His housekeeper told the court that he had privately confided in her, revealing that he regularly took the drug throughout the day, using it before he ventured out anywhere, resorting to it when he was 'irritated', and at night when he needed to sleep. She herself had occasionally been called on to give him his dose when he went to bed and she stated that 'he had acquired the practice of swallowing large doses ... a tablespoon at a time'. By the close of 1825, according to her privileged knowledge, he had been purchasing forty-nine grains of solid opium and one ounce of laudanum daily. During the two years before the Earl's death those who knew him had observed gradual changes in his habits, in that he became increasingly gloomy, low in spirits and neglectful of himself. His friends believed that the prospect of financial ruin was the only cause of his decline but it was, unknown to them, accompanied by an increased consumption of laudanum of up to three ounces per day.[20]

17 Christison, *Cases and Observations in Medical Jurisprudence*, pp.132-3.

18 Ibid., p.659.

19 Ibid., p.123.

20 Ibid., pp.126-7. See Appendix 1 for dosages and strengths.

The discreet behaviour on the part of the 'better ranks' of opium-eaters reveals the desire or need for secrecy. For the Earl of Mar it may have been a sense of shame, particularly in his last years, both at his impending ruin and his increasing dependency on opium that drove him to hide himself away. Physician's apparent reluctance to divulge knowledge and experience of opium-eating may also have stemmed from this sense of shame. Compared with the other professions medicine was not held in high regard. Its inadequacy in the face of disease and death was obvious to all and its dealings in the corruption of the flesh tainted it with disgust, immodesty, and disrepute. The new areas of medical specialisation that were emerging at this time often appeared implicated in the vices that were responsible for the diseases.[21]

To a man the medical witnesses called upon in the Mar case - Drs Abercrombie, Duncan, Alison, Maclagan and Christison, and the surgeon-apothecary Mr Macfarlan - agreed that the habit of opium-eating 'must tend to injure the health and shorten life' but, nonetheless they also all stated, or admitted, 'that they had scarcely any direct experience in the matter'. Only Macfarlan was able to say he knew of someone with such a habit, a woman who had used about two ounces of laudanum daily for many years, and who had died at the age of sixty, though he could not recall the cause of her death. In court Christison had divulged the circumstances of a number of similar cases which, he said, had been communicated to him by 'a friend'. This information, he conceded, 'tended to show, that opium-eaters may reach a fair age' but he still thought that, as a moderate dose was known to cause digestive disorder, so it 'must generally injure the health and shorten life'. Accordingly, and assuring his readers of his impartial and 'dispassionate' view of the facts, Christison could not agree with the decision of the judge and jury that the insurance company was liable. In his opinion the Earl's life had been proved to be 'clearly hazardous' and the judge had not been sufficiently well acquainted with the long-term effects of the habit. The 'special fact' of the Earl's ability to consume a tablespoon, that is half an ounce of laudanum at a time, and that this did not appear to be an unusual dose for him, testified to the excessive extent of his habit. Christison was adamant that 'no one could safely swallow this quantity, which is six times the largest and twelve times the ordinary medicinal dose for unaccustomed persons, without the long and frequent practice of using it in gradually increasing doses'.[22]

It was clear to Christison that the widely held notions about the 'peculiar effects of the opium-eater's dose' were largely based on the sensational, romantic, and vague statements of those who had travelled in the East. He also thought that most medical men had been erroneously influenced by these tales, for they were deluded that opium would merely throw an individual 'into a state like the excitement of intoxication from wine or spirits ... to remove dullness and depression'.[23] Further, he wrote, 'it is in consequence supposed that in general much excitement is in the

21 R. Porter and G.S. Rousseau, eds, *Sexual Underworlds of the Enlightenment* (1987), p.206.

22 Christison, 'Case X. On the effects of Opium-eating', pp.126-7.

23 Christison, 'Of the Action of Opium', pp.645-63.

first instance produced, in the midst of which every individual yields himself up to extravagant acts and expressions, corresponding with his ruling passions'. Christison noted an experiment with opium made by one of his colleagues, relating that 'if in the evening when he felt sleepy, he took thirty drops of laudanum, he was enlivened so that he could resume his studies; and if, when the usual drowsiness approached, which it did in 2 hours, he took a hundred drops more, he soon became so much exhilarated, that he was compelled to laugh and sing and dance'. This gentleman was reported as having 'repeatedly made the experiment' leading us to acknowledge the possibility that the pursuit of empirical science was not his only motivation.[24]

Christison himself was convinced by his own observations and experiences that such effects must be extremely rare. Whilst he was inclined to think that those unaccustomed to using opium might experience 'tranquillity and brilliancy of ideas', they could also fall prey to many 'disagreeable idiosyncratic effects'. According to his rational account 'the state of the opium-eater, while under his dose, is not at all different from that of an ordinary person of active habits, cheerful disposition, and liveliness of ideas [and] in many instances, when an opium-eater is under the influence of the drug, no one could possibly have any suspicion of the fact'. That there was a desire to conceal the habit, even from close acquaintances, Christison partially explained by describing the 'gloom' and 'depression' that followed the 'state of elevation' which drove the opium-eater to 'take care not to be seen at that time'. Should meeting others be unavoidable the user could always 'alter the face of matters by renewing his dose'.[25] The professor did not, however, offer any greater insight into what impulse or sensibility may have compelled the user to hide away from society. The opaque, romantic depictions of the consequences of opium use as related by eastern travellers were roundly dismissed in favour of 'medical materialism'. This term was first used in the eighteenth century to describe the manner in which religious or visionary experiences were explained away as being due to drugs or even digestive disorders.[26] Coleridge had put it thus: 'Doctors are *shallow* animals; having always employed their minds about Body and Gut, they imagine that in the whole system of things there is nothing but Gut and Body'.[27]

The medical profession, attempting to interpret and confine esoteric experiences within an objective and measurably empiric system, was typified in Christison's 'appeal to special facts'. He had been unable to discover 'any facts of the least value on the subject in medical records', so he supplied experiences related to him by several of his friends on whom he felt he could rely for their verisimilitude. These were disclosed as follows:

24 Ibid., p.649.

25 Ibid., pp.134-5.

26 M. Douglas, *Purity and Danger: An Analysis of the Concepts of Pollution and Taboo* (1966), p.33.

27 Coleridge, letter to Charles Lloyd, Sr, 14 November 1796, in E.L. Griggs, ed., *Collected Letters of Samuel Taylor Coleridge* (1956), I, p.256.

1.
A young lady of five-and-twenty has taken it largely for fifteen years. It was first administered secretly by her nurse to keep her quiet and save trouble; and the unhappy lady was subsequently compelled to keep up the practice for her comfort. She enjoys good health.
2.
A female, a patient of mine in the Infirmary, a martyr to rheumatism, took it for ten years previous to her fortieth year in the quantity of a drachm daily of solid opium. She then gave it up. Six months afterwards she was attacked with jaundice; subsequently she was several times severely ill of rheumatism; and she died in her forty-third year of consumption. This woman, however, led a licentious life from an early period.
3.
A well-known literary gentleman who has taken laudanum with some intermissions for twenty years, and occasionally to the extent of nine or ten ounces daily, has now attained his forty-fifth year. He is in spare form, looks older than he is, but is capable of undergoing a good deal of bodily fatigue, and enjoys tolerably good health so long as he takes sufficient exercise. His allowance when I last had an opportunity of conversing with him was about nine drachms of laudanum daily.
4.
A lady in this city, after drinking laudanum to excess for upwards of twenty years, died about the age of fifty. No information could be supplied about the disease of which she died.
5.
A lady of the same age takes about three ounces daily, and has used it for many years. She appears to enjoy good health.
6.
A lady, about sixty years of age, has taken it above twenty years, and is in good health.
7.
A charwoman, who had been in the daily practice of drinking two ounces of laudanum for many years, died at the age of sixty. The gentleman who stated this fact, does not remember what disease she died of, although he dissected the dead body.
8.
An eminent literary gentleman, I am informed, has been in the habit of taking laudanum since he was fifteen; and his daily allowance has sometimes been a quart bottle (twenty-six ounces) consisting of three parts laudanum and one of alcohol. Enormous as this dose may appear, I am assured the fact is well-known to his acquaintances. He is about sixty years of age, and enjoys good health.
9.
A lady of seventy, now alive, has taken about half an ounce of laudanum daily for nearly forty years. She enjoys tolerable health, and every year travels great distances to her friends.
10.
An old woman of eighty died a few years ago at Leith, after taking about half an ounce of laudanum daily for nearly forty years; and she enjoyed tolerable health all the time.[28]

Christison realised the inherent contradictions in his work, not least he knew that opium-eaters with a chronic habit might attain a good age, but still he persisted in his belief that it was inimical to a long life. To explain this he conjectured that

28 Christison, *Cases and Observations in Medical Jurisprudence*, pp.132-3.

it was more than probable that many people died at an early age of the effects of opium-eating, 'before their secret is detected'. The 'parallel fact' that 'drunkards' were also often long lived did not in his opinion bear out the conclusion that drunkenness was favourable to longevity. Indeed, he fully anticipated that the habit of opium-eating would eventually be found to be just as destructive as 'the vice of drinking spirits'.[29] 'The general impression', Christison concluded, was that the practice 'injures the health and shortens the life', but he wisely warned against the possibility that 'the scientific physician in modern times [should] allow himself to be hastily carried along in the present instance by vague general belief'. His use of the phrase 'scientific physician in modern times' reveals the medical profession's need for cultural validation, and informs the argument for the creation of addiction as a disease entity.

The *bête noire* that addiction would become had its public debut as a social menace in anxieties about poisonous substances. The burgeoning medical profession, through its journals and in the national press, aired its concerns over this lack of knowledge and control of drugs. The more coverage there was, the greater the ignorance revealed, and the keener the profession was to rectify and inform. The beginnings of the debate on poisons soon had physicians and their patients enthralled.

Suicide, accidental poisoning, and the growing response

> *He who makes a beast of himself gets rid of the pain of being a man.*
>
> Samuel Johnson

Poisoning was a common way of committing suicide throughout the nineteenth century.[30] As Christison had remarked in his *Treatise on Poisons* (1829), opium was often sought out by the timid for this purpose because of the gentleness of its operation. Its use was not a new phenomenon, but it was becoming more of a concern alongside the general anxieties surrounding the issue of poisons. The distinction between medicine and poison, between self-medication and self-destruction, was always, as we have seen, equivocal. No one could be sure that a solitary death brought about by opiates was accidental or deliberate, unless accompanied by some definite evidence that pointed to suicide. The doubts and difficulties were manifold in a time

29 Ibid., pp.133-4. For the perceived relationship between opium and alcohol see Appendix 2.

30 Suicide with opiates has a long history. Hellenistic and Roman peoples certainly employed opium, a drug overdose being a common means of ending one's life '*cum valetudo inpetilibus odium vitae fecessit* (when an unbearable disease had rendered life hateful)'. Pliny described such deaths, including that of the father of Publius Licinius Caecina, a senator c. AD 68-9, '*item plerosque alios* (and thus also several others)', in J. Scarborough, 'The opium poppy in Hellenistic and Roman medicine', in Porter and Teich, *Drugs and Narcotics*, pp.4-23.

when widely available opiates were the most effective analgesics and offered both physical and mental solace, when the quality and strength of the drug could vary so greatly from preparation to preparation, and when individual tolerance was rarely taken into account. Those who were habitual users might also go to their deaths with opium, but their intentions often remained unclear.

Cases of successful and failed suicides, for example, along with the attending physician's reports, were appearing in the *Edinburgh Medical and Surgical Journal*, as early as the 1820s. William Howison, Fellow of the Royal College of Surgeons, Edinburgh, wrote in that journal in January 1822, 'On the Medical and Moral Treatment of Young Women who have swallowed Laudanum in large Quantity, with a design of proving fatal to Life; illustrated by two Cases successfully treated'. The two young women, aged seventeen and eighteen, had both been disappointed in love but their cases presented Howison with 'little interest', and worse, 'no novelty'. They were considered unique neither in their misery nor in their physical recoveries which were 'mainly attributable to the usual and well-known means – the production of vomiting, exposure to the air, and keeping up a state of motion of the body, to obviate the strong tendency to stupor'. The moralistic attitude to what the physician called the young women's 'mistaken shame', and their '*nefarious practice*' of swallowing laudanum, also aroused negligible professional interest at that time, being roundly and decisively dismissed as being 'very commonplace'.[31]

Much of this behaviour came to light through inquest cases such as Mary Inge's, first reported in the local *Kentish Observer* and later picked up by the *Times* in August 1834. She was a young married woman found lying dead in a hop-pole stack, clutching in her hand her last bottle of laudanum. Mary had spent the last three months of her life in Westgate gaol and had died early on the morning of her second day of freedom. Her inquest was held at the Eight Bells in St Dunstan's, Kent, and before the coroner a witness called Harriet Wellard deposed that Mary had left the gaol in 'perfect health', carrying the sum of 5s 6d which she, Harriet, had given her. She also revealed that Mary had been one who 'habitually took opium', but that she had 'taken no opium during her confinement' in Westgate. The surgeon who was providing the inquest with medical evidence gave it as his opinion that, 'from the condition of the pupils of the eyes ... and the absence of all marks of violence', Mary had suffered an overdose of the narcotic. For, he said, 'by suspending the use of opium for the time alluded to, a person could certainly not take the same dose as when in the habit of taking it', and that the quantity of the drug he had found in her body 'was sufficient to destroy life'. Mary could not have been sure of the quality nor the measure of opium she had bought, for her laudanum would have been made up on his premises by the individual druggist. The report concluded with the statement, 'The Jury, after a patient investigation, returned a verdict - "That the deceased died from having taken opium, but not with intent to destroy herself"'.[32]

---

31 *Edinburgh Medical and Surgical Journal*, 1822, 3, p.29.

32 *Times*, 5 August 1834, p.3, col.e, 'Death From An Overdose Of Opium', reprinted from the *Kentish Observer*.

So what was Mary's intent? What needs or desires had sent her to her final dose of this draught? Was she ill or depraved, perhaps she was deeply miserable, merely foolish, or maybe just seeking some pleasure and comfort? Whether any of these questions were asked, or any possible answers given, was not deemed of sufficient importance to be included in the report. Although Mary may have begun to use opium for medicinal purposes, as many lifelong users said they did, had she been sick whilst in gaol she would almost certainly have been given some of this ubiquitous palliative, for the institutional use of opium was widely accepted.[33] We know that she had been accustomed to taking opium and must assume that she had been without her drug for some weeks whilst incarcerated. Free to take it again, she had perhaps misjudged the dose or had simply not been aware that her tolerance level would have fallen. Perhaps she was celebrating her release, or even facilitating it with a blissful oblivion. What the short, bleak story of her accidental death provokes in us is a curiosity about the use, and the meaning of the use, of opiates. From the detached, almost disinterested tone of the press report this was at the time, it seems, a commonplace pursuit, largely hidden perhaps because of its very unremarkable familiarity. This apparent acceptance was of an unorthodox, non-medicinal use of opium.

Such cases became familiar to readers of the medical journals and the national press, and were undoubtedly informative in a shared practical sense. At half past three on the afternoon of 16 June 1839, Caroline Mercy, a young married woman of thirty-two, was taken to the Manchester Royal Infirmary in a state of complete insensibility, having attempted to poison herself. James Harrison, a physician who assisted with the case, later wrote to *The Lancet* relating the 'novelty' of the resuscitation techniques employed and the collective 'feelings of astonishment' which were evident at the success of these ministrations. What was described as Caroline's 'moral history' was retailed to illuminate the case, showing how doctors assimilated and responded to their patient's experiences, psychological as well as physiological.

Caroline's husband was a master-plumber who had failed in business and was reduced for a number of years to living 'irregularly'. She had left him after two years of distress and dejection, returning to the comfort her mother offered. Foolishly believing his ardent promises of amendment she went back to the plumber, but was all too soon disappointed and felt too ashamed to return again to her mother. The couple quarrelled violently, Caroline left the house and running to four different shops she purchased sixpennyworth of laudanum at each, receiving about a dessert-spoonful for every penny. She swallowed down each measure as she got her hands

33 Many long-term users of opium said they had, or were said to have, begun their habit through medicinal necessity: see for example Berridge and Edwards, *Opium*, pp.70, 212; Hayter, *Opium and the Romantic Imagination*, pp.27, 165, 191, 226, 255; *Times*, 23 March 1894, p.9, col.e. The institutional use of opium was as widely accepted as general use for most of the nineteenth century: see for example A. Scull, *Museums of Madness* (1979), pp.170, 203; *Times*, 21 January 1848, p.7, col.e; 4 July 1867, p.11, col.b.

on it. At the Infirmary, where the distraught and now stupefied young woman was taken by a neighbour, her medical attendant began his repertoire of treatments. Her hair was pulled, her skin was pinched, she was doused with a sudden affusion of icy water. Putting her to bed, Mr Samuel Gaskell, then Superintendent of the County Asylum at Lancaster, had introduced the stomach-pump with a gallon of cold water but thought it prudent to desist as his patient's condition deteriorated. Still he felt he had to try once more, and injected two ounces of liquid ammonia in about as many quarts of water. As her condition gradually worsened he applied large sinapsisms, or mustard plasters, down the length of her back and, with what must have been an increasing sense of desperation, began to pour boiling water over her arms, legs and feet. A full hour after her admission Caroline's breathing was noted as being 'very considerably embarrassed; the inspirations and expirations being separated by unusually long intervals' and Dr Gaskell, believing the young woman to be about to die, 'thought it desirable to assist the respiration by artificial means'. The two men stood each side of Caroline and 'alternately raised and depressed the ribs, in imitation of customary actions'. They applied ammonia to her nostrils and forcibly struck her face and chest with a wet towel. After two hours, during which time if the doctors ceased their work she relapsed, Caroline raised her eyelids. Her ribs were 'everted', most probably broken, the skin on her chest was raw and bloody and she had been severely scalded by the boiling water. So essential, so intrinsic to the medical practitioner's therapeutic art was opium, that for her wounds and to sedate her Caroline was prescribed, every night until her discharge nearly two months later, twenty drops of laudanum, the agent of her physical tribulations. This treatment was noted without any acknowledgment of irony. There was simply no alternative.[34]

It is apparent that for their poisoned adult patients, medical practitioners having, if possible, ascertained how much of the drug had been taken and when, would then proceed to run through a gamut of possible remedies. This continued until either one or another of their ministrations appeared to have effect or until they lost their

34 Present-day management of acute poisoning with opioid analgesics usually involves the intravenous administration of Naxolone, a specific pharmacological antagonist. There are complications with the use of this drug in opiate addicts as it may precipitate the distress of acute withdrawal syndrome. It may also make the addict's behaviour 'troublesome' if their intoxication is fully reversed and they insist on leaving medical care before the risk of lapsing back into CNS (central nervous system) depression has disappeared. Controlled trials have indicated that gastric emptying does not significantly alter the course of poisoning and only in a minority of cases are toxicologically important quantities of drugs recovered. Gastric lavage may even increase the severity of poisoning by forcing toxin through the opening of the stomach into the intestines and enhancing absorption. Emetics (such as Impecacuanha) are not harmless either as vomiting may persist long after the period when poison might be ejected thus delaying the beneficial administration of charcoal. The trend now is towards abandoning gastric lavage and induced emesis in mild and moderate poisoning and replacing them with repeated doses of oral activated charcoal which can more easily absorb the amounts being retrieved. See A.T. Proudfoot, *Acute Poisoning: Diagnosis and Management* (1993), pp.17, 34-5, 164-5.

patient, perhaps when he or she 'merely forgot to breathe'. There are numerous accounts of the stimulating administrations of emetics such as zinc oxide, of warm baths and sprinkling with cold water, tickling and pinching, continual walking up and down, shaving the head, dextrous use of the newly patented stomach-pumps, and, by the 1840s, electricity and electro-magnetism.[35]

Called upon to resuscitate the potential suicide, the physician was engaged in a desperate and often violent life and death struggle and, whilst the nature of these situations cannot be denied, the treatments could be interpreted as carrying harshly punitive elements. A note in the 'Medical News' section of the *Lancet* in the 1850s was entitled 'The Stomach-Pump a Punishment' and it reported that an apothecary in Ireland was paid 7s 6d to administer it.[36] In later years, with the benefit of hindsight and the construction of disease theory, the eminent physician Sir Clifford Allbutt gave it as his opinion that early remedies had been as useless as they were barbarous. The catalogue of their efforts indicate a need and a willingness to try literally anything, however specious, in order that this knowledge, or a 'cure', might be forthcoming.

Cases such as Caroline's were by no means rare and were extensively related and discussed within the pages of the journals. Another case given detailed attention was that of a nineteen-year-old girl, also suffering from opium poisoning, who was brought by the police to the Islington workhouse at eight-thirty on the night of 11 March 1841. She had procured an ounce and a half of laudanum and had drunk all of it an hour and a half before her admission. She was lucid enough to tell the surgeon brought to attend her that the cause of her attempted suicide was seduction. She begged him to allow her to die. The doctor's response was to administer a drachm of sulphate of zinc 'which caused her to vomit freely ... the stomach-pump was then employed, and a large quantity of warm water was injected into the stomach: this fluid was then withdrawn, and the contents of the stomach completely evacuated'. Next, and 'not withstanding her remonstrances', she was taken outside into the cold night air and, supported by two men, was compelled to walk the yard incessantly. She begged to be left alone but the doctor insisted she be 'literally dragged about'. Despite her relapse into torpor the unfortunate girl was 'freely' fed strong coffee, a 'solution of ammonia was held to the nostrils, her ears were tickled with a feather, and she was pinched and shaken ... for nearly two hours'. Her ordeal continued through this long night with mustard poultices being applied to her calves 'which excited great irritation', until four in the morning when she began to recover her sensibilities. The account ends abruptly with the note that 'in a few days she became free of all unpleasant symptoms' and the surgeon felt able to discharge her, pronouncing her 'cured'.[37] Physicians agreed that it was necessary physically to rid the body's system of the drug and to ensure constant and often vigorous stimulation

35 See for example *Lancet*, 1824, 1, p.375; 1824, 3, p.173; 1825, 6, p.157; 1826, 8, pp.191, 381; 1834, 1, p.258; 1836-37, 2, pp.354-9; 1838-39, 2, pp.924-7; 1840-41, 1, pp.190-2; 1843-44, 1, pp.572-4.

36 Ibid., 1853, 1, p.282.

37 Ibid., 1840-1, 1, pp.190-2; 1840-1, 2, pp.186-7.

to prevent those suffering an opium overdose from sinking into stupor and death. But it is also clear from the reports, into the mid-century and beyond, that there was no definitive medical knowledge of the actions of the drug and how it might affect an individual.

The journal reports of experimentation and experience were supplemented by statistics of poisoning which begin to appear from the late 1830s and were taken from the returns of coroner's inquisitions. One such compilation of statistics, which appeared in the *Edinburgh Medical and Surgical Journal* in 1840, was broken down into counties and the types of poisons resorted to. The article includes the emotive and sympathetic statement that the information 'is fraught with deep and melancholy interest'. Recognising this, the *Gateshead Observer* had 'reduced the returns into a compact and popular shape' so that the 'public may be benefited', perhaps by having their sensibilities and anxieties aroused, but also to be warned of carelessness in the use of familiar but potentially harmful substances.[38] In the latter account brief descriptions of the reasons behind the deaths are given and it is pertinent to note here that of the two most popular drugs used, accidental deaths from overdoses of arsenic comprised about 10 per cent but deaths from opium consumption were 50 per cent of the total number. Opium, as has been said, was the only effective analgesic available for most of the nineteenth century and it was in constant common use, whereas arsenic was not administered in the same fashion, as we shall see. The varying strengths of the imported opium and the marked differences in the individual druggists' preparations, discussed elsewhere in this study, in conjunction with the guesswork which accompanied self-administration, were generally recognised to be the root cause of accidental poisonings.

The increasing levels of interest on the part of the medical profession and the public revealed by these articles illuminate the emerging awareness of the extent of everyday drug use and its real and perceived dangers. The terminology of 'harm' and 'risk' applied to attitudes towards unorthodox drug use was also to be found in emerging public health ideology. Edwin Chadwick referred to the use of opium when speaking to the inquiry into drunkenness in 1834, and he reiterated his concerns in his *Report on the Sanitary Condition of the Labouring Population* in 1842.[39] A letter published in the *Lancet* in 1840 appealed to public-minded sentiments in requesting assistance with inquiries 'into the use and employment of opium in health and disease'. The correspondent particularly asked for information regarding the 'correctness of the various reports relative to the increased consumption of opium by the upper and lower classes of society', revealing not only the growing search for answers but also how social and moral values were increasingly concerned by the consumption of the drug.[40]

---

38 See for example *Lancet*, 1839-40, 1, pp.597-9; *Edinburgh Medical and Surgical Journal*, 1840, 53, pp.256-64.

39 P.P. 1842, XXVII: *On the Sanitary Condition of the Labouring Population*: Local Reports for England and Wales, 3, p.212.

40 *Lancet*, 1840-1, 1, p.423.

These concerns about opium use were discussed at a meeting of the Royal Medical and Chirurgical Society on 24 November 1840, following a paper entitled 'Observations on the Improper Use of Opium in England'.[41] The speaker, Julius Jeffreys, stated that he wished to elaborate on the 'great and alarming increase ... of opium-eating in England, and to solicit from the Society some declaration which might have the effect of discouraging such practice'. The term 'opium-eating' had come into common parlance with the publication of De Quincey's *Confessions* in 1821, and if it provided a recognised cultural reference point, it may also have added an undesirably populist flavour to this paper from which the physicians present may have wished to dissociate themselves.

Jeffreys depended for his evidence on the customs house returns of the quantity of the drug imported into England each year between 1820 and 1838, 'by which it would appear that a very considerable increase had been experienced'. Whereas the quantity entered for home consumption in 1820 was found to have totalled 16,169lbs, the figure for 1838 had risen dramatically to 131,204lbs, an eight-fold increase in less than twenty years. Responses to the paper were, however, decidedly guarded. The anonymous reviewer noted that this increase was something which merely 'appeared' to the author to be of growing concern, thus expressing some cynicism on the part of most members of the Society who were present. Three physicians gave it as their opinion that the increased consumption was to be explained by the increase in population, by the drug's being more frequently used than it had previously been, and by 'the greater frequency of late years of those maladies in which opium is employed'. They obviously wished to emphasise orthodox use and to avoid the suggestion of 'luxurious' use and any implication of medical responsibility for its apparent increase.

Much of the audience was anxious to make it plain that in their opinion opium 'was used more as an anodyne than as a stimulant, even in those who did resort to it habitually', that there was little opium-eating among the poor patients admitted at major London hospitals, and that dispensary patients very rarely used the drug as a luxury. One Dr Ashwell remarked that he had made 'accurate inquiries' in some large manufacturing towns on the question of increased consumption among the 'poorer inhabitants', and stated that he had found no such increase taking place as was described in the paper that evening. Some of the physicians spoke of their doubts about offering any 'decided opinion' on the improper use of opium and thought that 'indeed, harm might be done' should any resolution on the subject be passed. The Society members present reiterated the great importance of keeping knowledge of the drug within the medical profession, reminding each other of Sydenham's emphatic statement that he would have given up the practice of medicine if opium were to be expunged from the pharmacopoeia. Keen to maximise its respectable therapeutic role and to play down its luxurious one, their wish to avoid any resolution being passed suggests that they regarded the latter to be inherently dangerous, outside any real understanding or control, and that they believed that acknowledging the

41 Ibid., pp.382-3.

purely stimulant effects would serve to reveal this and might encourage 'improper' consumption. They were particularly concerned about such use amongst the poor, implying that these people were regarded as the more susceptible, hence weaker, strata of society and that the educated physician had a growing duty to protect them from the misuse of a drug which should remain firmly in the province of his profession.

Despite these concerns, one or two of their number chose to digress. A Dr Webster believed that both in London and in the country 'opium-eating was carried on to a great extent', but that 'being a secret vice it was difficult of detection'. Others, in comparing opium-eating to gin-drinking, remarked that they considered the latter to be the more harmful to the individual and to society as a whole. One physician went so far as to say that if he had to choose between the two he would prefer the use of opium for it 'had not the incentives to the commission of crimes' and, further, it 'could never demoralize the habits and shorten life, as gin-drinking did'.[42]

In the 1840s, attempting to quantify numbers of suicidal deaths from poisoning, William Farr, the pioneering and dynamic first statistical head of the General Register Office, had argued that they could be substantially reduced if drugs for medicinal purposes were obtainable only on prescription, and those used in the 'arts and manufactures' only on presentation of an official certificate. Farr believed that 'in certain states the mind appears fascinated ... by the presence of a fatal instrument', and that 'the withdrawal of the means of death suffices to save lives'.[43] Even though the medical profession and those involved in public health believed that restriction was the best way to prevent what they understood as this misuse of drugs, there was little effective legislation during the nineteenth century.

But by 1855 the *Lancet*, in a piece on medical jurisprudence, considered these deaths were becoming far *too* commonplace. The article detailed the suicide statistics of the records of the Western Division of Middlesex for the years 1852 to 1854, and was intended for the use of the medical profession and the advantage of the community. The chosen district was inhabited by 'upwards of *nine hundred thousand* human beings' and included many important suburbs of the metropolis, several of the country's most important hospitals, five railway lines, and numerous charitable institutions, asylums, workhouses, and industrial establishments. Of the total figure of 2,674 inquests held, 216, or 'rather more than one-twelfth of the whole number' were suicides, and this figure comprised 'only those cases in which suicide was clearly proved, and not instances in which persons were found in water, &c., ... where a doubt existed whether self-destruction had been committed'. Of the proven suicides thirty-two were recorded as self-poisonings.[44] Between 1863 and 1882 opiates were the most popular of suicidal poisons for women and the second most favoured amongst men, and by 1907 the fourth for women and the third for men.[45]

---

42 See Appendix 2 on the perceived relationship between opium and alcohol.

43 *Lancet*, 1841, 1, p.101.

44 Ibid., 1855, 1, p.47.

45 O. Anderson, *Suicide in Victorian and Edwardian England* (1987), p.366, n.89.

The journals and popular press carried leaders on the 'numerous cases of attempted self-destruction' by poison, and these were often cited in support of the growing and pressing argument against the indiscriminate sale of poisons. One such article in the *Lancet* considered that many a suicide acted upon an impulsive moment, 'intoxicated, as it were, by some apparently calamitous provocation, added to their uncontrolled passions or morbidly sensitive minds'. An obstacle, such as legislation, placed in the way of a potential suicide could be sufficient to allow 'successful remonstrance of the voice of the conscience', and a terrible disaster might be averted. As many such deaths were considered to be the result of fleeting or overwhelming passions, stemming perhaps from jealousy or disappointed ambition, it was thought that it might be enough merely to remove the immediate means. The 'ineffectual' suicide would not then be tempted to try again, or at the very least, he or she might adopt some other, less controversial, method of self-destruction. The author illustrated his argument with the case of an officer's widow who had cut her own throat after 'having previously taken sufficient opium to have caused death', and with three recent charges against young women who had attempted to kill themselves with poison over some 'trifling circumstances'. These 'unfortunate and misguided beings', who were numbered amongst the 'excessive' accidental and criminal poisonings, could, he thought, have been spared if the sale of poisons was not, with the exception of arsenic, utterly unrestricted by law. 'Why', he asked, 'should opium ... and such like, be as easily and freely obtained as the common necessities of life?'[46]

These fears were emphasised by reports such as that of the 'lower class of women', admitted to the parochial infirmaries to give birth, who took opium with 'impunity'. These young mothers secreted beneath their pillows 'a phial of laudanum or a box of opium pills ... put there for daily use', and freely spoke to each other of their 'favourite druggist shops' where they might get a better measure than elsewhere.[47] A physician picking up and commenting on this 'habitual consumption of opium amongst the [lower] class' believed that it occurred to a 'far greater extent than is generally supposed by the public'.[48] And however much this gentleman might have imagined or wished opium-taking to be a lower-class habit, it seems that much of the 'public' from all social strata were more familiar with the inclination to seek the particular pleasures of the drug than he supposed, and that the 'respectable' and the elite were also busy purchasing their 'halfpenneth of elevation'.[49]

The medical profession was caught in a cleft stick, encouraging and reporting scientific advances in pharmacology whilst wishing to prevent the enthusiastic, promiscuous, and unregulated use of new compounds. Newly patented preparations of opium constantly appeared in the medical marketplace and were often acclaimed

---

46 *Lancet*, 1852, 2, pp.334-5.

47 *Times*, 21 January 1848, p.7, col.e., from *Dr. Winslow's Journal of Psychological Medicine.*

48 H. and P. Coombs, eds, *Journal of a Somerset Rector 1803-1834* (1984), p.467.

49 Charles Kingsley, *Alton Locke* (1851).

in the medical journals and national press. Messrs Gale and Co., for example, wholesale chemists of 15, Bouverie Street, London, were commended in the *British Medical Journal* for their introduction of Opiatine, a combination of morphia and codeia, 'freed from the odorous and inert principles – the resin, oil and impurities of opium – and in which the active constituents are in an uniform, concentrated, and reliable condition'.[50] But, whilst the outcry about the unrestricted sale of poisons continued, letters appeared in the journals arguing that to 'restrict a chemist from selling poisons would be equivalent to ordering him to close his shop at once'. Such a move was a nonsense, it was argued, for what would become of the 'bird-stuffers, the straw-cleaners, the boot-makers, the braziers, and all that class of artisan whose work depends on such drugs?' And if the druggists were to be so served then, 'by the same rule, all sellers of knives and forks, and guns and pistols, ought to be extinguished too'.[51]

The Sale of Poisons and Pharmacy Act of 1868 had a limited effect on the situation. A 'Schedule of Poisons' was established which called for all substances on the list to be clearly and fully labelled and sold only by registered pharmacists. For the poisons in Part I of the schedule the prospective purchaser had to be known, or have been introduced, to the pharmacist and all details of the sale, including the date, the quantity sold, the reason for purchase, and the name and address of the purchaser and his or her sponsor were to be recorded in a Poisons Register. This pattern of sale, enforceable or not, was adhered to for the next forty years and changes were made only when agitation by manufacturers, shopkeepers and dealers called for a free trade in poisons, ostensibly to provide for the farming community. The legislation, and eventually the 1908 Act which ended the pharmacist's monopoly over some specific poisons in common use, failed significantly to reduce accidental and homicidal poisonings and had even less effect in reducing suicidal poisonings.[52] It was always argued that a superficially calm but determinedly suicidal person could easily purchase his or her chosen drug and that the clearly labelled 'Poison' bottle, even if previously bought for a legitimate household purpose, might actually suggest a means to an end for a potential suicide.[53] So ubiquitous and familiar was opium as a household medicinal standby, that it remained a favourite with suicides even into the early twentieth century.

The campaign for restrictions on the sale of poisons amongst the medical profession was attended by powerful and emotive statements on the perceived abuse of drugs by the layperson and by those whom they saw as unqualified to deal in such potentially dangerous substances. 'Week after week, and almost day after day',

50 *British Medical Journal*, 3 March 1877, p.270.

51 *Lancet*, 1850, 1, p.195.

52 Berridge and Edwards, *Opium*, p.121. The accidental opium death rate declined very slightly from the pre-restriction level of c. 4 per million population but remained at between 3 and 4 per million until the 1890s. The opiate suicide rate showed very little variation until the 1890s when carbolic acid replaced it as the poison of choice.

53 Anderson, *Suicide*, pp.362-5.

the *Lancet* regaled its readers with 'the recorded cases that point the necessity of more stringent measures to check the indiscriminate sale of poisonous substances'. Legislation was stridently demanded to prevent those 'unconscionable scoundrels who dare to tamper with human life by administering medicines of whose properties they are grossly ignorant, for diseases they know nothing whatever about'.[54] Again in 1858 the *Lancet* printed one of many articles on the 'Poison Shops' which 'constantly added to the list of those murdered by the careless sale of poisons'. It criticised the local papers which reported the incidents as though they were singular events. They were singular 'only in their unusual atrocity: in the more than ordinarily blind ignorance of the vendor, his criminal carelessness, and double-dyed stupidity: they are not singular in any other respect, but repeat in painful monotony the features of a dozen cases'.[55] In 1858, in a discussion of the Sale of Poisons Act, the *Lancet* was cynical but enthusiastic. It suggested that the proposed restrictions were 'so severe that either they will be practically disregarded ... or they will amount to a virtual prohibition of the sale of these poisonous substances to the general public ... a thing by no means to be deplored'. The author of the editorial estimated that 'one hundred and twenty persons may ... be supposed to die annually in England' from opiate poisoning. But, worse, how many, he asked, are 'slowly killed by the pernicious and terrible habit of opium-eating ?'[56]

He suggested that this practice was increasing to an enormous extent. People were driven to it as a 'mild and certain means of death, when life has become intolerable' and, deplorably, as a common 'intoxicant'. Opium had been 'placed kindly within their reach by an indulgent Legislature'.[57] Twenty years later the *British Medical Journal* published a piece on the 'Free Trade in Poisons' and was still emphasising the 'necessity for some strong legal restrictions on the sale of poisons'. 'Scarcely a week passes', it read, 'without reports of inquests on the bodies of persons who have fallen victims to this kind of free trade'. Despite the necessity of recording the details of any sale it was not illegal to sell twenty bottles of poison to one customer, and coroners strongly condemned the 'mock legislation' which 'practically legalise[d] the sale of a ready instrument' for suicide, murder or for 'voluntary poisoning ... by the pernicious habit of opium-eating'.[58]

An inquest on a 'Man Unknown' conducted at Westminster in November 1861 heard that a labourer found dead from an overdose had long been in the habit of taking laudanum and had sent his girl out for more to help him sleep. In the absence of any other evidence it was merely recorded that he had 'died from the effects of an overdose of laudanum'.[59] A near-fatal case of opiate poisoning in an habitual user was described in the *British Medical Journal* in 1866 and was attributed by the victim

---

54 *Lancet*, 25 April 1857, 1, p.435.
55 Ibid., 15 May 1858, 1, p.486.
56 Ibid., 17 July 1858, 2, pp.69-70.
57 Ibid.
58 *British Medical Journal*, 27 January 1877, p.115; 31 August 1867, p.179.
59 Anderson, *Suicide*, p.230.

as being due to a 'better quality [of laudanum] than that which he usually drank'. In an attempt to revive him the unfortunate man was subjected to the stomach pump, pinching and pricking with needles, and was endlessly walked around. Finally he was slapped sharply with wet towels, exhausting the several policemen brought in to assist and entirely destroying the four new reel-towels used in the process.[60]

This is not to say that, although death from opiate poisoning might be one of the gentler routes into the afterlife, it was necessarily the easiest. One Samuel Hillier, paymaster-general in the Ninth Lancers, left behind a suicide note in 1860 in which he declared himself to be almost 'poison-proof'. 'About ten days ago', he wrote, 'I took half an ounce of laudanum, enough to poison a horse. It had no effect on me. After that I took eight grains of opium, again no effect, except a slight drowsiness. Then four grains of morphia; no effect. I then took five grains of liquor opii sedativus, with the same result'. This determined but disappointed character was eventually reduced to shooting himself.[61]

Poisonous fears and poisonous years

The *Pictorial Times* of Saturday 4 December 1847 uncompromisingly declared the mid-nineteenth century to be the 'Poisoning Aera'. The *Lancet*, in November 1858, claimed in tones quivering with barely contained hysteria that, 'it is terrible, this invasion of poison. Our homes are assuredly no castles, but dens of horrid device, where we are surrounded by cunningly-wrought instruments of death and disease'. These publications were not alone in making their startling claim. The metaphor of poison and its attendant anxieties resonated, ever more strongly, through Victorian culture, slowly seeping into the public consciousness with a subtle, pathogenic ease.[62]

Accounts of deliberate and accidental poisonings were frequently to be found in the pages of newspapers and medical journals during the mid-nineteenth century. The *Times* carried many such tragic and disturbing stories, both as a form of fascinating if morbid entertainment and as a public-spirited warning.[63] Undoubtedly, an awareness of potential harm, perceived and actual, was nurtured amongst the public. Like a culture in a petrie dish, it was a silent, stealthy, infectious and malevolent growth.

The inquest of Ann Kirkbride reported in the *Times* in 1854 also reveals a casual, everyday use of the drug. Ann was a child of 22 months whose mother 'had been accustomed to chew opium' and had been 'in the habit of buying [it] by pennyworths at a time'. Whilst playing the girl had discovered 'about one third of that quantity in

---

60 *British Medical Journal*, 7 July 1866, pp.15-16.

61 Berridge and Edwards, *Opium*, p.81.

62 M. Harris, 'Social Diseases? Crime and medicine in the Victorian press', in W.F. Bynum, S. Locke, and R. Porter, eds, *Medical Journals and Medical Knowledge: Historical Essays* (1992), pp.108-125.

63 See, for example, the *Times*, 20 May 1857, p.10, col.d; 10 October 1860, p.9, col. a; 14 August 1863, p.12, col.d; 16 December 1872, p.4, col.f.

a can' left by her mother and had consumed it, dying in hospital the following day despite recourse to the 'usual remedies to cause the ejection of the narcotic'. Ann was described by the press 'An Infantine Opium Eater' but there was no comment, moral or otherwise, in the report on her death of her mother's daily use of the drug. This was ignored by the paper and once more raises the question as to whether the woman's habit was considered remarkable at all. It would appear not. In another press report of the same year William Merrill, aged thirteen years, was billed as 'A Youthful Opium Eater' when he came before Kettering petty sessions charged with obtaining goods and cash under false pretences. It was reported that 'the lad was reared by his grandmother, now between 80 and 90 years old [and] an inveterate opium eater', who had given her grandson the drug 'ever since he was a month old'.[64] Infant doping with proprietary medicines and self-medication with laudanum and opium pills was, as has been suggested, both usual and considered necessary. Accidental deaths due to overdosing on opiates were occasionally reported in the press and by the mid- to late nineteenth century were exploited by factions lobbying for tighter control over poisons.[65]

The pervasive taint of poison can be almost tangibly detected in the *Lancet* articles of the period. A near-fatal accidental poisoning was detailed in July 1855 which unusually offered the victim's own account of his experience, deemed to be quite as valid and informative as the attending surgeon's remarks on his prescribed treatments. Francis K-, aged nineteen, had mistakenly received the wrong compound from a druggist shop in Glasgow, and in order not to waste any of what he believed was a 'precious medicine' he had 'washed the physic-basin twice and drank the contents thereof'. His ensuing experience gave a personal and quite visceral quality to the medical case history. He felt 'immediately (in his own words) as if a powerful electric shock had passed through his head – he expected that his brains would have burst through his skull'. A similar case reported in April 1856 provoked the attending physician categorically to state that the problem of poisoning was becoming 'rife'. To give weight to his opinion he listed six recent cases ranging from a gentleman 'hurried in to eternity by the wanton carelessness or culpable negligence of two boys employed in the dispensing of drugs, of whose nature or properties they are grossly ignorant', to three others poisoned by the 'stupidity of a servant giving aconite root for horseradish', and a husband who 'cunningly removes an encumbrance, in the shape of a wife, by strychnine'.[66]

Alongside the ubiquitous reports of suicides, accidental poisonings and the celebrated mid-nineteenth-century trials of the likes of Dr William Palmer, 'the Rugeley Poisoner', there appeared the sordid exploits and tales of those who lived

64 *Times*, 25 August 1854, p.5, col.f.

65 Such tragedies still occur today and even now, despite strict controls, they are sometimes iatrogenically induced. An inquest in the *Independent* on 28 January 1997 related the 'unnatural death' of a baby girl in a neo-natal intensive care unit who was injected with more than 100 times the required dose of morphine.

66 *Lancet*, 1855, 2, pp. 52-3; 1856, 1, p.369.

amongst, or ventured into, the sort of company recorded in *Blackwood's Magazine* in 1856. It carried a flagrantly baroque account of 'A Recent Confession of an Opium-Eater' which was subsequently reprinted in the *Times* as 'An Opium-Eater Among Burkers'. The article had all the sensational ingredients of a ripping tabloid exposé, with sex, drugs, one-upmanship and a narrow escape from a fearful and sordid death. The brave narrator purported to be 'studying the aspect of humanity in the Rembrandt-like chiaroscuro of vice and crime'. In search of the 'harmonies which slumber in the soul of man' he had 'sounded the base string of society', thereby acknowledging the weaknesses within all men and allowing his readers to shudder at the potential poison within themselves. The story began in a 'dingy chamber in the topmost flat of a many-storied and ancient dwelling' in Edinburgh where the narrator had become engaged in a drinking competition. It was not long before he realised that his miscreant hosts intended to 'hocuss' him in some dire way. Unknown to the conspirators, the narrator had a habit of consuming a pint and a half of laudanum *per diem*, and was able to quaff the laudanum he was given glass for glass with his opponent's port.[67] He felt himself to be a monument to, and a triumph of, opium-eating, a sort of semi-respectable and controlled user, not a raddled addict, and in every way superior to his companions. The port-drinker, 'Long-nosed Bill', who possessed a remarkably villainous physiognomy, became 'confused, and [was] no longer master of his utterance', whilst our 'hero' became 'calmer and calmer and flow[ed] on in a rapt strain of eloquence' that afforded him 'immeasurable delight'. But, with incipient horror, an awareness of some 'unutterable malignity' stole over him as he became alive to his situation. Feigning a stupefied collapse he watched Bill and his woman totter to another room where there was a bed with two mattresses, a 'complication of ropes, pulleys and weights, and a sack'. Realisation dawned. 'Heaven and earth', he silently exclaimed, for he had heard of such things before: 'the unhappy being, stupefied by opium, is placed between two mattresses and smothered, so as to produce the appearance of a natural death, and his body sold to surgeons'. Our hero was in the company of 'burkers', and was about to be 'burked' himself. Whilst their backs were turned to their victim he stealthily filled their port glasses from his bottle of laudanum and was ready to face them, 'seated upright and cheerfully surveying them'. So astonished were they at his apparent recovery that they agreed to continue drinking the health of the lady with their miraculous guest. Eventually, as their muscles relaxed, their heads sank to their chests, their breathing deepened, and they fell side by side on the floor, our hero reflected on their insensibility, and on 'the train of symptoms by which they who dare trespass, without the initiation and neophytism, on the imperial domains of opium'. Our intrepid narrator left.

Even allowing for journalistic verve and elaboration, the subject of this cautionary tale was already a very real concern, so much so that it had formed a

67 One and a half pints of laudanum would equate with approximately 4.5 grams of morphine meaning that the narrator had a heavy drug habit. See Appendix 1 for doses and relative strengths.

clause in the 1851 Act for the Better Prevention of Offences. The legislation recommended imprisonment and transportation for those sufficiently wicked to use 'any chloroform, laudanum, or other stupefying or overpowering Drug' to facilitate a robbery or any form of attack on others. In 1861 the Offences Against the Person Act also included the felonious use of laudanum in an attempt to deter any such crimes. It is impossible to estimate any effect these provisions may have had on the criminal use of opiates as the Registrar General's calculations did not take into account the use of the drugs merely temporarily to stupefy. It has been argued that the official lack of comment on this crime suggested that it was, and perhaps never had been, of any great importance, but it would be more pertinent to point to its very intangibility as a reason for any such bureaucratic silence.[68]

Arsenic poisoning, deliberate and accidental, was also a source of much anxiety amongst the medical and legal professions, as well as with the general public. The *Lancet* considered that the 'habitual employment' of arsenic 'complicated a hundredfold the already bewildering difficulties of toxicology in its juridical relations', engendering such questions as 'how to convict of arsenical poisoning when ladies use arsenical cosmetics [and] when confectioners sell arsenical sweetmeats?'[69] This particular potent compound received so much attention that an Arsenic Act was passed in 1851 to restrict the unorthodox use of the drug. The Act declared that the unrestricted supply and sale of the drug facilitated the commission of crime, and it intended that particulars of every sale should be entered into a book before the arsenic was handed over the counter. These criteria included the purpose for which the drug was required, the vendor's signature, and the name, address and occupation of the purchaser, plus a witness's details if the purchaser was unknown to the vendor. Further, arsenic was to be sold only to adults and to be coloured by mixing it with soot or indigo. Any person selling an unauthorised preparation, or discovered giving false information to obtain it, would be 'summarily convicted before magistrates [and] be liable to a penalty not exceeding £20'.[70]

But still the nefarious use of arsenic continued, as demonstrated and reported in a poisoning case brought before the Edinburgh courts in 1857. Madeleine Smith, described as 'handsome, accomplished … religious and respectable' had become 'physically debauched', dragged into 'lower moral depravity', and finally stood accused of attempting to poison her paramour. Her saviour was Christison. He argued that the quantity of arsenic in the dead man's stomach was too great to have been secretly administered without his realising it. This expert opinion was morally enforced by the defence claim that such a woman would never have risked exposure by resorting to murder.[71]

68 Berridge and Edwards, *Opium*, p.82.

69 *Lancet*, 'Arsenic for the Million', 1860, 2, p.592.

70 Ibid., 1851, 1, p.312; S.W.F. Holloway, 'The regulation of the supply of drugs in Britain before 1868', in Porter and Teich, *Drugs and Narcotics*, pp.77-96.

71 Madeleine had been surreptitiously introduced to the young man and had received his advances, allowing him to seduce her despite her parent's opposition. She began writing

A leader in the *Lancet* two years later stated that, although the legislature had done its best to hinder the illicit use of arsenic, it seemed that the effect had merely been to induce 'a resort to other poisons rather than to diminish their frequency'. More worryingly, it alleged that manufacturers and tradesmen seemed to be doing their best to 'nullify the benevolent intentions of the Legislature in protecting us from the criminal administration of arsenic by substituting slow and ingenious processes of domestic poisoning, and introducing such a quantity … into articles of home use as may readily supply the fatal dose'. The author asked his complacently unsuspecting reader to imagine sitting 'unconscious in his library, on a summer day, his walls coated with arsenic, a suspicious green dust on his books ... it fills the air … gets into our food, poisons our bread, or mayhap, as orpiment, adds a fatal charm to our "Bath buns"'. Scheele's green, or arsenite of copper, possessed the 'fatal gift of beauty in its combinations', surrounding and haunting the Victorians in their socks, paints, tapers, lampshades, and who knew what other apparently harmless everyday article. As well as 'impregnating all the air with fine arsenical dust' it seemed that the very atmosphere was fraught with, and poisoned by, a general and public insecurity. 'Nothing', the author despairingly concluded, 'is innocent now in this world'.[72]

The reader of such frightening pieces was advised to learn to expect, or to 'see' poison, as 'Adam was fated to see the serpent hidden beneath the leafy cover of the tree of knowledge'. He or she was now subject to all manner of scares, including, for example, the 'Death in the Snuff-Box', wherein the *Lancet* had fearlessly tracked 'the Destroyer … in his most secret haunts'. In this instance analysts had discovered that in the lead linings of snuffboxes 'a chemical action is excited which has the effect of charging the snuff with sub-acetate of lead'.[73]

It was a mark of how very ubiquitous these reports and scares had become that they began to be the subjects of parody. On 4 December 1858 the *Lancet*, not normally regarded as a satirical oasis, reported on the horror produced in Paris by the alleged planting of poisonous trees along the city's Boulevards. It was said that, should a single drop of the sap from these, interestingly, 'Chinese' trees fall upon the bare skin, 'the most venomous ulcers [would] arise – ulcers which are incurable, and end in the painful death of the victim'. Those 'savans of renown' who were putting the scare-story about reported 'the care with which the promenaders avoid

obscene letters to her lover whilst encouraging the advances of yet another suitor. While she blew hot and cold, her first lover began to suffer the symptoms of arsenic poisoning and eventually died a sordid and violent death. The dead man was scathingly portrayed in court as a 'miserable little fop … of inferior station … a vain and impulsive little coxcomb' in the habit of plastering his face with arsenical cosmetics to enhance his complexion. He had, in consequence, already suffered deleterious effects from the self-administered poison, as well as having twice previously attempted suicide: 'the attribute of a coward', according to the defence. The jury then proceeded to acquit Madeleine of murder, despite her having bought arsenic before visiting her lover on the night of his death and openly, in the presence of respectable witnesses, told a deliberate lie as to why she wanted it.

72 *Lancet*, 'Medical Annotations', 1860, 1, pp.149-50.

73 Ibid.

either walking or sitting in the shade of these "arbres maudets"'. How gullible, how impressionable to poisonous anxieties, had the general public become, educated as they now were to fear and even to abhor their very environment.[74]

Toxicology: the need to define poison

Sad mechanic exercise,
Like dull narcotics

Alfred Lord Tennyson, *In Memoriam*, v, 1869

Popular fears of poison, once encouraged and expressed, demanded explanation, and were they both placated and exacerbated by the pronouncements of toxicology. In the preface to his major taxonomic work, *On Poisons in Relation to Medical Jurisprudence and Medicine*, Alfred Swaine Taylor, toxicologist and first Professor of Medical Jurisprudence in Guy's Hospital, London, concurred with the view of the national and medical press that the mid-nineteenth century was an era soaked in poison.[75] First published in 1848, his medico-legal study ran through many editions and came to be valued by lawyers and physicians alike as the standard work on the subject during the remainder of the century.[76] Taylor was a renowned expert on toxicology, on the absorption, deposition, elimination, detection, and classification of poisons, and his studies are still published today by his successors at Guy's. He achieved a formidable reputation in his field and 'performed an invaluable service in codifying legal precedents and rulings and relevant anatomical and chemical data'.[77] Regularly employed in the courts for the defence and the prosecution, any poisoning case to which he lent his expertise was recognised as being both serious and celebrated. His name became increasingly familiar in the national press as well as in the medical journals. Consequently neither he nor his profession escaped controversy, particularly during the infamous William Palmer, or 'Rugeley', poisoning case tried at the Old Bailey in 1856. Taylor's biographical entry in *Munk's Roll* portrays him as 'a commanding figure in the witness box, unbending and relentless', but both his rigid manner and expertise came under attack by observers such as the social commentator Henry Mayhew. On the publication of Mayhew's interview with Taylor during the Palmer trial there ensued an undignified journalistic spat in the *Times* and the *Daily*

---

74 Ibid., 1858, 2, p.348; 1858, 2, p.575.

75 G.H. Brown, ed., *Munk's Roll: Lives of the Fellows of the Royal College of Physicians of London 1826-1925* (1955), 4, pp.73-4. A.S. Taylor, 1806-80, received his education at Guy's and St. Thomas' Medical School and in Paris under the leading toxicologist, Orfila. In 1831 he was appointed to the newly established chair at Guy's and held that position until 1877.

76 Taylor's other works, equally revered, include *Elements of Medical Jurisprudence* (1836) and forming the basis of *A Manual of Medical Jurisprudence* (1844); *On Poisons in Relation to Medical Jurisprudence and Medicine* (1848); *The Principles and Practice of Medical Jurisprudence* (1865).

77 Brown, *Munk's Roll*, pp.73-4.

Telegraph.[78] Taylor complained that the interview had been obtained surreptitiously and was nothing but a scurrilous parody of his true words. He most fervently denied having remarked that, should he have been a secret poisoner himself, he would have given his victims sufficient poison 'before [he] had done with them'. The whole sordid episode was, he thought, all 'perfectly disgraceful' and gratuitous, but it was a worryingly unfortunate brush with the arrogance of science and did little to raise public confidence in the poison experts.[79]

The case was probably the most celebrated of the century and was reported in great detail in the daily and the medical press. William Palmer, thirty-four years old in 1855, had been a licensed general practitioner in Rugeley, Staffordshire for some ten years. A series of financial disasters centering on the racetrack were alleviated by his collecting £13,000 in insurance money on the death of his young wife. Following swiftly on this first family tragedy, a second substantial amount then arrived on the death of his brother, and, lastly, one of his creditors suffered a suspicious demise. Palmer maintained to the steps of the gallows that he was innocent of the poisonings. The prosecution called Taylor as the expert medical witness and the case ignited a grand controversy over evidence and, in particular, the infallibility of medical knowledge. According to some press reports, Taylor and his peers had abandoned their 'positions as indifferent auxiliaries of justice' and 'advanced pretensions to direct and administer it'. If this was so, they argued, it would be impossible:

> for the ordinary administrators of the law to test a skilled witness, who becomes, in fact, himself, a sole jury, whose verdict is the more fatal, inasmuch as, however he may be led astray by the fantasies of science, the instinct of the chase, or the influence of popular prejudice, he is commonly a man of unquestionable respectability, and often of considerable talents of learning.[80]

In 1857 Taylor and toxicology were again under attack, this time by the medical profession itself in the pages of the *Lancet*. At an inquest in Stamford, Taylor had allegedly 'proceeded to examine the medical witnesses precisely as a barrister would have done; subsequently stating his own opinion on the evidence elicited, and concluding by a most un-called-for judgement on the opinions expressed by one of the medical witnesses'. He had, it was thought, assumed an entirely arrogant and inappropriate 'double duty'; medical knowledge, as Christison had declared in 1851, was constructed from observation and opinion and was therefore fundamentally at odds with the need for legal 'facts'. The resulting imbroglios, rather than conveying a professional confidence to the already insecure public mind, further fanned the anxieties about poison and perfidy and left belief in the discipline of toxicology in shaky esteem.

78 B. Harris, 'Social Diseases? Crime and Medicine in the Victorian Press', in Bynum, Lock, and Porter, *Medical Journals and Medical Knowledge*, pp.108-25.

79 Ibid., p.116

80 I.A. Burney, 'A poisoning of no substance: the trials of medico-legal proof in mid-Victorian England', *Journal of British Studies*, 1999, 38, 1, pp.59-92.

Poisoning cases such as William Palmer's provided increasing amounts of sensational column inches for the daily press. The publication of a 'Rugeley Number' by the *Illustrated Times* was rumoured to have doubled that paper's sales to 400,000. *Punch* suggested that the 'Poisoning Cases' had been, a 'delicious hope for the paragraph-mongers, who have been literally living upon poison for nearly a month'. The *Daily Telegraph* invited its readers to imagine what could be 'more wonderful than that a drop of clear liquid … should still all that subtle machinery of life in a moment. One convulsive shudder, and the brain … will cease to think, the senses to feel, the heart to beat, and the limbs to move!'[81] The enigmatic and terrifyingly intimate nature of poison was intended to infect, and perhaps thrill, the public imagination. The *Times* indulged a *frisson* of panic in a leader on 22 August 1859, and, discussing another of the infamous poisoning trials of the mid-century, the writer speculatively asked his enthralled readers:

> Who can hope to penetrate into the mysteries of this great town? Who can tell what is passing in any one of the dull uniform rows of houses of which London is made up? The true history of a single street would be a more romantic chronicle than any which the novelist has conjured up.

The *Lancet*, too, in an article in 1855 chillingly entitled 'Poisoner in the House', played on the anxieties and titillated the fancies of its audience, bringing the threat right into their homes and amongst their loved ones. 'If you feel a deadly sensation within', it warned, 'and grow gradually weaker, how do you know that you are not poisoned? If your hands tingle do you not fancy that it is [poison]? How can you be sure that it is not?' One of the most insistent medical journals to cover this perceived threat was the *London Medical Gazette*. Published under Taylor's editorship from 1845 to 1851, it carried a long series entitled 'On the Increase of Secret Poisoning'.[82]

'Poisoning' was then, and still remains, an emotive term and as such it has required close definition within the scientific and legal communities. In his preface to *On Poisons in Relation to Medical Jurisprudence and Medicine*, Taylor was at pains simply to emphasise the 'fearful' increase in poisoning, the rapid pace of progress in toxicology and, especially, the 'comprehensive nature' of this 'distinct science'. It was, he believed, a body of research and knowledge necessary not only to the course of justice but also to the very security of the individual and of society as a whole. He speculated, in the broadest of fashions, that there was probably 'no branch of medicine in which we meet with a larger assemblage of truths … combined under one common character'. Thus he re-emphasised the seemingly total permeation of poison throughout society together with the validity of a science that could describe all manner of aetiologies, symptoms and remedies.

But these were dangerously shifting semantic and pharmacological sands, and medical consensus struggled to gain factual *terra firma* with statements such as the

81 Ibid., pp.119, 121.

82 Ibid., p.67 n.25, 70.

following, made in 1855: 'A virulent poison may differ from the most wholesome food only in the difference of quantity of the very same ingredients'. And only 'in popular language' was a poisonous effect thought to result from a small quantity.[83] Twenty years later the debate was alive and well within the pages of the *British Medical Journal*. In an article entitled 'Legal Administration of Poison: What is a Noxious Substance?', the journal discussed a case in which the defendant was accused of administering a noxious compound to a young woman 'with intent to excite the sexual passion, in order that he might have connection with her'. The trial turned on the argument as to whether 'the term "noxious" depended on quantity as well as on the nature of the substance'. The prisoner was found guilty of 'intent to injure, aggrieve, and annoy', but was acquitted because he had given his victim only a small amount of the drug. The journal was outraged; it damned the evidence of the 'incompetent and inexperienced witness' and argued that such an offence should anyway carry penal consequences. The credibility of the medical profession could not be called into question by allowing such dubious results, and noxiousness could not be allowed to rest solely upon an indefinite condition of quantity. If it was, the writer argued, 'we do not see how it is possible to suppress ... poisoning'.[84]

In 1885, mindful of the shared interest of medicine and the law in drugs, *The Encyclopaedia Britannica* was still bemoaning the fact that an exact definition of 'poison' was by no means easy: 'there is no legal definition of what constitutes a poison'.[85] The earliest references to these medico-legal concerns related to the responsibilities of physicians, rather than to any contribution medicine had made to legal knowledge.[86] Under British law there is still no explicit legal definition of 'poison'; it remains understood as 'any destructing or noxious thing' that may be 'employed with intent to murder, to enable an indictable offence to be committed, to endanger life or inflict grievous bodily harm, or to injure, aggrieve or annoy'. So

83 OED, 2nd edition.

84 *British Medical Journal*, 24 March 1877, pp.358-9.

85 J. Stevenson, in *The Encyclopaedia Brittannica*, xix, 275/2. The 2nd edition of the *Oxford English Dictionary* defines poison as 'any substance which, when introduced into or absorbed by a living organism, destroys life or injures health, irrespective of mechanical means or direct thermal changes'. This is now further qualified by three components: firstly the poison, which might be any substance derived from mineral, plant, animal, or synthetic origin; secondly, the route into a living system, regardless of how simple or elaborate that may be; and thirdly, that there be an adverse response. Only when these components are fulfilled can poisoning be said to have occurred; though in the absence of one of them it might be suspected, Walton, Beeson, and Bodley Scott, *The Oxford Companion to Medicine*, 2, pp.1113-14.

86 Walton, Beeson, and Bodley Scott, *The Oxford Companion to Medicine*, 1, pp.396-7. The earliest references are found in the Babylonian Code of Hammurabi where the rights and duties of physicians are detailed. The lists include penalties for medical negligence, abortion, wounding and poisoning. Inevitably medical procedures carry legal implications and in this sense medical jurisprudence was and is regarded as encompassing all of medical practice.

that even though certain specified substances are statutorily scheduled as poisons and their manufacture, distribution, sale and supply are regulated, this does not necessarily mean that all these compounds are universally harmful, nor that any which are unregulated are without deleterious effects. It is understood that any inherent harmfulness will vary widely between one substance and another, that the effects on an individual will differ depending on size, sex, and other physical and mental qualities, and that fatal quantities will alter according to the method of administration, i.e. oral, dermal, by injection, or by inhalation.[87]

Taylor had provided a common definition of poison as any substance 'which, when administered in small quantity, is capable of acting deleteriously on the body'.[88] But this, he remarked, was 'too restricted' a definition, for it excluded a very substantial class of materials which had undeniable poisonous properties but which would only prove deleterious in larger doses. The notion of '*quantity* ... therefore [could not] be made a ground for distinguishing [the] poisonous from [the] non-poisonous'. Here his views were in accordance with his contemporaries who were also struggling to define the point at which a food might become a poison and *vice versa.* They were searching for a point of distinction between a beneficial and a detrimental effect.

In an article published in 1851 in the *Edinburgh Medical Review* Christison had written of the mutability of medical 'facts'. The science of medicine, he argued, rested on 'opinion' and this in turn had its foundation in 'observation', which rendered it heavily subjective as well as nominally objective. The general public was required to merely accept medical opinion, differing as it did from physician to physician, and laced as it may have been with subjective cultural prejudices. Furthermore, the law, in particular, was faced with a fundamental mismatching of method.[89] Under the law 'a question of fact left for the decision of a jury' was taken 'from the medical evidence given in the case', and, in order to avoid any technical objection, an indictment generally contained a clause describing an offending substance as a poison or '*noxious thing*'. So, as Taylor admitted, medical witnesses were 'severely pressed in cross-examination on trials for certain criminal offences, to state', despite all the scientific ambiguity, 'what is strictly a poison and what is not'.[90]

In terms of medical jurisprudence, Taylor had stated again and again the difficulties inherent in providing 'such a definition of a poison as shall be entirely free from objection'. He could only offer, as 'perhaps' the best suggestion, that it should be understood as 'a substance which, when taken internally, is capable of destroying life without acting mechanically on the system'. But objections remained, for if a substance were applied to the body externally and caused injury or death but did not act in a 'purely mechanical' manner, would that substance not then be a poison too, even though it be boiling or icy water, for example? Even if swallowed these

87 Ibid., 2, p.1114

88 A.S. Taylor, *On Poisons in Relation to Medical Jurisprudence and Medicine* (1848), p.1.

89 Burney, 'A poisoning of no substance', pp.83-4, n.75.

90 Taylor, *On Poisons*, pp.4-5.

substances could not be said to act mechanically, but would nonetheless injure or kill due to shock to the nervous system, yet, surely 'it would be inconsistent to class these inert liquids among poisons?' If they were so classified then the 'whole class of medicines, and numerous substances of an inert nature, would be included', and such a system would obviously be untenable. Any distinction in medico-legal terms, Taylor therefore asserted, should not even be attempted 'except by a professional man, who has given attention to the subject of toxicology'.[91]

Today the accumulation of technique and instrumentation allows the detection of the minutest deposits of alien substances in the human body. However, there still remains the enigma of whether any such compound may have acted pathogenically or not: that is, a distinction must be drawn between what might be expected or commonly found and what might be a dangerous excess, either self-administered or possibly present through sinister misdeed. It is still common for authorities to offer contradictory and conflicting views, especially in the course of legal hearings.[92] It is now also accepted that the side effects of therapeutic doses of drugs are also seen as manifestations of poisonings, to the extent that there is an independent discipline dealing with such adverse reactions. Thus clinical toxicology is now concerned with excessive doses of drugs, or substances not intended for ingestion, inhalation, or application to the body; the introduction into the body of chemically inert substances that obstruct internal passages causing deleterious symptoms are also regarded as poisons. Where the taking of drugs is non-medical, or 'illicit', it is of greater pertinence to note that it is now thought that 'exposures which do not cause unwelcome and adverse consequences, whether experienced by the individual or identified in him or her by others, are not "poisonings"'. 'Illicit' drug taking is now less emotively described as 'non-toxic exposure'.[93] Neither Taylor nor his colleagues made any similar distinctions, replete with sub-agenda of deliberate self-poisoning or drug taking for pleasure, in the mid-nineteenth century.

The most eminent authorities on toxicology in our period understood poison in the broadest and most comprehensive of terms. Taylor and his colleagues still concurred with Paracelsus who, four centuries earlier, had unequivocally stated that 'all substances are poisons; there is none which is not a poison'.

Concluding remarks

The actual and metaphorical notions of poison as a source of fear and disgust were thus gradually emphasised and accepted by the mid-Victorians, who came to perceive themselves as living in an insecure world thoroughly permeated with the poisonous. They were already familiar with newspaper accounts of deadly poisons

91 Taylor, *On Poisons*, pp.7-9.

92 Walton, Beeson, and Bodley Scott, *Oxford Companion to Medicine*, 2, p.1114.

93 Proudfoot, *Acute Poisoning*, p.1. The commonest form of poisoning now, among adults, is deliberate self-poisoning, accounting for at least 95 per cent of all such admissions to hospital.

lurking in everyday domestic objects, with the debate over adulteration of food and drugs, deliberate and accidental poisonings, drug suicides, and the sordid or romantic tales of habitual opium-eaters. These accounts acted as a focus for unspecified anxieties about pollution, and portrayed a subtle, corrupting permeation of society and the individual by the unseen and the unwholesome. The everyday familiarity with drugs such as opium became tinged with less than subtle doubts about their use and poisoning was increasingly being recognised as 'peculiarly the crime of civilisation'.[94] And if this were not seen as danger enough, what was society to make of those who actively chose to poison themselves, some to the extent that they could not live without their noxious substance? The apparently voluntary self-poisoning of drug addiction was increasingly perceived as unorthodox, alien, shameful, and fraught with danger, if not as yet a crime.

94 Burney, 'A poisoning of no substance', p.67 n.25, 70.

Chapter Six

Observation and Experience: The Enquiries of Medicine into Addiction

He labelled and he libelled this and that,
The genus and the order,
And wiped his feet on Nature's temple mat
But did not pass the border.

With book and scale and speculum and probe
He burrowed, measured, minimized, and crawled
From patch to patch by details yet enthralled,
And but beheld the shadows of the globe.

For mind and matter were to him but one
And bundles of sensation,
Or states of feeling vanishing, and none
Had any true foundation.

Frederick William Orde Ward, 'The Scientist',
English Roses (1899), Section III, 'Laughing Philosophy'

Background to changes in the medical perception of addiction

This chapter centres on the abundance of eighteenth-, nineteenth-, and early twentieth-century medical treatises and case histories that trace the development of medical opinion on addiction. A chronological reading of these works can be seen, starkly, as a journey from a generous interrelationship of ideas to a more specific, unforgiving and mechanistic understanding. But, despite the functionality of much of the argument, as the debate flourished the condition was increasingly embellished with symbolism. It became full of meaning for the drug users and those around them, clouding a purely scientific and empirical explanation despite the proclaimed faith of some contributors in the possibility of impartial clarification and their desire to provide it.

As the medical profession attempted to bring opium under its controlling auspices during the nineteenth century, the drug and its properties were increasingly discussed and thought of in purely medical terms. It inevitably followed that a disease concept of addiction, where a particular aetiology and certain symptoms were seen to occur, would emerge. The idea that addiction was a disease entity came into ascendancy riding on the coat-tails of the 'rise of science', and the new scientific model of addiction enhanced, and served to entrench, a moral view of opium users.

The perception of addiction as a pathological condition arose as it was increasingly harnessed to diseases of the nervous system, specifically of the will and as a form of insanity. The traditional theory of disease was derived from classical humoralism, a system which remained the dominant theoretical basis for diagnosis and treatment well into the nineteenth century.[1] In this holistic model 'dis-ease' was seen as a lack of harmony and balance in the four basic 'humoral elements' of the body: blood, phlegm, black bile and yellow bile.[2] Any imbalance would be the result of immoderate living, imprudent passions, and a poor health regime. Belief in the unity of mind and body convinced physicians that they had the ability to understand and treat disturbances of the mind and that they were not concerned with somatic sickness alone.

In the eighteenth century the work of Georg Ernst Stahl brought a proto-psychology into medicine. He argued that all the basic phenomena of life were governed by the 'soul', and that through this agency the reciprocal relationships of the 'passions, or mental reactions, and the accompanying organic changes could be explained'.[3] Any disturbances in the mind were the result of an abnormal relationship between the mind and the body. In the 1790s Erasmus Darwin had posited a system of nervous reflexes which reconciled soma and psyche. Describing a 'continuum of stimuli leading from elemental physical irritations, up through sensations and volitions, to the association of ideas', he argued that psychological disturbances might have a physiological root.[4] Addiction, or the recognised state of 'enthralment', could then also be viewed as something internally, rather than externally caused: a condition involuntarily acquired rather than voluntarily induced, and one that might be cured by the proper application of medical science.[5] The late eighteenth- and early nineteenth-century emphasis on nervous pathology firmly linked mental and physical illnesses to one another and provided an explanation of the interplay between organic life and consciousness. Mainstream somatic medicine, laying emphasis on cellular pathology, could then suggest that brain cells were 'the agents of all that is called mind'. A 'physiological psychology' developed, making a valid addition to what constituted a scientific explanation, and which came within the growing cultural authority of science.[6] This was the foundation on which the later identification of addiction with nervous diseases, hereditary conditions, and moral insanity rested.

1 V.A. Sharpe and A.I. Faden, *Medical Harm: Historical, Conceptual, and Ethical Dimensions of Iatrogenic Illness* (1998), p.38.

2 The two humors thought responsible for madness were yellow and black bile. The former was hot and dry and caused irritation and inflammation leading to mania or frenzy; whilst the latter was cold, dry, thick and sour, and caused melancholy.

3 I. Veith, *Hysteria: The History of a Disease* (1965), p.187.

4 R. Porter, *Mind-Forg'd Manacles*, p.179.

5 R. Porter, 'The Drinking Man's Disease: "The Pre-History" of Alcoholism in Georgian Britain', *British Journal of Addiction*, 1985, 80, pp.385-396.

6 Scull, *The Most Solitary of Afflictions*, pp.184, 225, 238.

Addiction as a discrete disease entity also developed alongside the nineteenth-century drive for professionalisation by medical men. It was a symptom of the desire to differentiate between orthodox and unorthodox healers, and to make distinct the division between traditional medieval ways and modern scientific medicine. The 'so-called' age of medical reform, recognised as a period stretching from the late seventeenth to the twentieth century, encompassed this process and was unrelenting and often vitriolic, rich in accusation and counter-accusation.[7] Before the Apothecaries Act of 1815 and the medical registration measures of 1858 there were no precise parameters to the term 'qualified medical practitioner', and the struggle for status inevitably included the designation and categorisation of the sick and of disease in order to legitimise the orthodox physician's claims. The controversy over the newly defined disease of addiction from the mid-nineteenth century onwards, and the attempts to control and regulate opiate use, were part of this process and were reflected in the medical texts and journals of the time.

Growing specialisation within the medical profession led to the rise of toxicology, to pharmaceutical developments, and eventually to the new sciences of neurology and psychology. The emergence and prevalence of the idea of addiction as a disease, specifically as a type of insanity and more often than not linked to hereditary causes, arose initially from the traditional duality of mind and body: the view that human nature was both somatopsychic and psychosomatic.[8] The emerging science of psychology was enlisted as part of the attempt to make the experience of addiction understandable in scientific terms. But, as advocates of psychological medicine were arguably fragmented, in as much as they were subject to the influence of the two new and quite separate disciplines of psychology and neurology, their efforts at empirical explanations of addiction seemed doomed. They appeared to be at worst inauthentic, and at least unsatisfactory, as they cut across boundaries of understanding and disciplines widely held to be contradictory.[9] An exploration of the developing debate within the medical profession is a pivotal means of understanding changing responses towards addiction and the uses of opium.

---

7 I. Loudon, 'The vile race of quacks with which this country is infected', in W.F. Bynum and R. Porter, eds, *Medical Fringe and Medical Orthodoxy* (1987), pp.106-28.

8 R. Porter, *Mind-Forg'd Manacles*, p.44.

9 M. Shepherd, 'Psychiatric Journals and the Evolution of Psychological Medicine' in W.F. Bynum, S. Lock, and R. Porter, eds, *Medical Journals and Medical Knowledge. Historical Essays* (1992), pp.188-206. As late as 1877, for example, the Senate of the University of Cambridge refused a proposal to introduce the study of experimental psychology because it would place 'the human soul in a pair of scales'. It wasn't until 1902 that the *Review of Neurology and Psychiatry* appeared, and explicitly stated the need to combine the disparate disciplines. The first issue included an introduction to the 'the steadily increasing conviction or the importance [of] the essential unity of the two subjects'.

Eighteenth- and early nineteenth-century writings on addiction

The possibility of finding oneself in a state of 'enthralment' to opium has been recognised since antiquity, but, because of the acknowledged beneficence of the drug, it had not, before the nineteenth century, been given great consideration. Addiction was, rather, seen as an unfortunate but necessary evil, and did not carry universal stigma. The properties and powers of the drug had traditionally been well documented and praised, and as a thaumaturgic palliative of the physician's pharmacopoeia and the lay person's experience, it was openly available and used by all. Even though there were very few doubts cast regarding its efficacy, some physicians were cautious: such a potent substance needed to be accorded respect.

Eighteenth-century medical texts constantly referred to opium as a thaumaturgic drug; indeed it was often viewed as a providential blessing of the 'Divine Architect'. In his work, *The Mysteries of Opium Reveal'd*, John Jones, a member of the Royal College of Physicians, described the effects of opium as akin to 'a most agreeable, pleasant, and charming Sensation ... seizing one not unlike the gentle, sweet *Deliquium* that we find upon our entrance into a most agreeable *Slumber*'. Moreover it was a 'delicious and extraordinary *Refreshment* of the spirits upon very good *News*, or any other great cause of *Joy*.' Jones had seen the wisdom of authoritative validation for his eulogy to opium by stating in 1700 that 'a Preparation of Opium stood [Paracelsus] in stead, and perform'd his Business when all his great Medicaments fail'd him; and that it will dissolve Diseases, as Fire does Snow.' It bestowed upon the user not only relief but also pleasant dreams, freedom from anxiety, release from pain, together with 'Promptitude, Serenity, Alacrity and Expediteness in Dispatching and Management of Business ... Assurance, Ovation of the Spirits, Courage, Contempt of Danger, and Magnanimity ... Euphory, or easie undergoing of all Labour, Journeys etc. ... Satisfaction, Acquiescence, Contentation, Equanimity etc.' Jones regarded it as 'indeed so unexpressibly fine and sweet a *Pleasure*', that it was very difficult for him adequately to describe it , 'or any to conceive it, but such as actually feel it ... therefore People do commonly call it a *heavenly Condition*, as if no *worldly Pleasure* was to be compar'd with it'. Such a heavenly condition did he consider it that, with true delight, and in a further effort to convey the drug's qualities he continued, 'it has been compar'd (not without good cause) to a permanent gentle *Degree* of that Pleasure which Modesty forbids the naming of'. And, he wrote, 'tis well worth a Remark, that both are *Pleasures* of the same Sense, *viz.* that of *Feeling*'.[10]

It is Jones's candid emphasis on the sensually pleasurable effects of opium that has earned him the criticism, not to say derision, of some twentieth-century scholars. Hayter, for example, attempting to describe the 'tradition' of opium use, refers to his work as 'an insidious misleading book [and] slightly mad'.[11] In this she reveals more of her own anachronisms and prejudices than any objective interpretation of the text, and she falls into the trap of discussing Jones as if he were deranged for elucidating

---

10 Jones, *The Mysteries of Opium Reveal'd* (1700), p.2.

11 Hayter, *Opium and the Romantic Imagination*, p.25.

his ideas on sensation. This too, it seems, became a 'tradition'. It is as though it has now been deemed in some quarters that the realm of the senses has no legitimate place in even a proto-scientific medical text; nor can the use of a drug for a non-medicinal purpose be seriously countenanced without accompanying judgemental comment. As Jones himself had noted, this very omission is one of the 'fundamental mistakes about *Opium* [and] one great *cause* why its *Operations* have puzzled and quite baffled all *Enquirers*', for they had 'gone upon a wrong Foundation in their Disquisitions'.[12] It is a return to these foundations, the sensory responses of those who took opium, which forms a major part of this book and helps to redefine the history of addiction.

Despite his eulogistic approach, Jones devoted a chapter of his work to a discussion of the possible ill-consequences of chronic opium use. In a chapter entitled 'The Effects of Sudden Leaving off the Use of Opium after a long, and lavish Use thereof', he attempted impartiality by explaining 'all its *Effects*' and 'seeming Contradictions' as he saw and experienced them.[13] Believing that the pleasure of opium 'is involuntary, and pleases us whether we will or no', he went on to describe '*Great, and even intolerable Distresses, Anxieties, and Depressions of Spirits*, which in a few *days* commonly end in a most miserable *Death*, attended with *strange Agonies*, unless Men return to the *Use* of *Opium*'. And what he called the 'inconveniences of leaving off' the drug, bore, he observed, 'a certain *Proportion* to the Time, and *Quantity*, that it has been used in', though he also maintained that 'The Mischiefs of excessive Doses, and lavish use [are] no *Argument* against their inspiriting *Nature*'. Indeed, even if you could not 'expect any *good Effects* from its *Excess*', then any ill-effects were 'not always to be imputed to the *viciousness* of the Thing used, but frequently of the *Person* that imprudently uses them'.[14]

Other eighteenth-century physicians investigating the consequences of taking opium regularly also knew very well what they were dealing with. They did not fail to remark upon the drug's obviously pleasurable qualities as well its pitfalls, and most were moved to censure 'luxurious' use for its evident dangers. Richard Blackmore, Royal Physician in Ordinary in the 1720s, though writing in praise of opium, was willing to confront the ill-consequences of 'wanton' or prolonged use:

> it is objected to the use of Opium, that, like Wine and Strong Liquors, it ... makes the Person sottish and stupid. I grant, that this is a frequent Effect of it, if taken wantonly upon small or no Motives, and that frequently, and that in an excessive Quantity: but no such pernicious Effects attend the use of it in a moderate Proportion.[15]

That opium could be habit-forming was a consequence he was familiar with and readily acknowledged:

12 Jones, *The Mysteries of Opium*, pp.23, 40.

13 Ibid., pp.33-4.

14 Ibid., pp.32, 85, 89, 238, 245.

15 R. Blackmore, *A Treatise of the Spleen and Vapours...* (1726), pp.83-9.

> Some Persons further object, that if they take Opiate Medicines, as they shall always be obliged to repeat them on the like Occasions, so Custom and Familiarity will so far weaken their Operation, that they shall be obliged to repeat the Quantity often, till at length they must rise to an immoderate Dose.[16]

The formation of an opium habit, in fact any habit, was, according to Blackmore, the responsibility of the user alone: the physician could not overcome what he considered the patient's predilection towards weakness. He wrote:

> I must acknowledge that some, for want of due Caution, or of Patience to bear small Sufferings, or a great Delight to keep themselves always easy ... indulge themselves too much in the use of Opiates ... as others have recourse too often to strong Wine ... and then it is no wonder if the one and the other by degrees contract such a prevalent Habit.[17]

Samuel Crumpe, in his *Inquiry into the Nature and Properties of Opium* (1793), also took pains to distinguish between the medical and 'luxurious' uses of opium, stressing that his own experiences were produced under experimental conditions to observe and discover the 'Effects of Opium on Living Systems'.[18] He had 'frequently and uniformly, experienced from large doses an increased flow of spirits, an observable gaity, cheerfulness, and alertness, which subsided into a state of pleasing langour'. These sensations were emphatically not comparable to the practice he saw as 'the solace of the wretched, and the daily source of intoxication to the debauchee'.[19] The physiological effects of opiates, including the possibility of addiction, were very familiar to physicians and were regularly discussed, though generally without the moral condemnation displayed by Crumpe, which, as we shall see, is more characteristic of the later nineteenth-century vilification of the drug.[20] As he pointedly remarked, 'almost every circumstance relating to this remarkable medicine has been the subject of dispute'.[21]

Crumpe's experiments and observations had shown him that when a regular user was deprived of his or her opium, even 'for a single day', they became 'languid, dejected, and uneasy at the customary hours of taking it, and could only be roused from this state by the usual quantity of Opium, or by a large draught of wine'. It is apparent that early medical opinions on opium addiction were based on observation and experience, on a straightforward appreciation of the drug, its effects and

---

16 Ibid.

17 Ibid.

18 Neil Vickers suggests that 'Crumpe's book seems to have had a strong influence on Coleridge', that he may have read it himself or read about it in the medical and literary periodicals. He did discuss it in correspondence with Southey, who had used it in his research for *Thabala the Destroyer.* N. Vickers, *Coleridge and the Doctors*, p.103.

19 S. Crumpe, *An Inquiry into the Nature and Properties of Opium* (1793), pp.22, 45, 48, 178.

20 R.B. Fisher and G.A. Christie, eds, *A Dictionary of Drugs* (1981), p.176; Harding, *Opium Addiction*, p.3.

21 Crumpe, *An Inquiry into the Nature and Properties of Opium*, p.11.

properties, and on the immutable knowledge that the drug was a vital part of the pharmacopoeia. It was also apparent that physicians believed that whether or not someone became an addict was consequent upon that person's strength of will.

Addiction as a disease

The formation of the disease entity of addiction was based on the question of will, on voluntary and involuntary reflexes which were a function of the nervous system. Nervous diseases or disturbances were themselves thought to have their origins in heredity, and, if sufficiently severe, were diagnosed as a form of insanity. Where addiction was concerned this was a 'moral insanity', a hybrid disease, a physiological affliction with behavioural symptoms that were open to judgement.

Debate over the effects of opiates, the controversies over their therapeutic use, and the disquiet over the possibility that they caused disease and insanity, was long-standing and full of controversy. Blackmore had lauded opium as an excellent curative for melancholy in 1726, George Young dismissed it as a useless remedy in 1730, William Battie, in 1758, believed it did a great deal of harm if improperly and freely administered, whilst Joseph Brandreth considered it nothing less than miraculous in 1791. In the mid-nineteenth century the arguments continued as, in the opinion of the Queen's physician, George Johnson, opium was so useful as to be recommended as a prophylactic, to be taken before any mental illness actually manifested itself. Some, such as Professor Johnston, recognised symptoms in the insane as analogous to the mental and physical phenomena experienced by opium users: 'without sleep and without food, restless as panthers, will not some maniacs show powers of endurance' such as could be seen amongst addicts? And, importantly, the 'influence of these narcotics resemble the workings of insanity [in] the weakening which they produce upon the Will'. In 1855 he argued that this form of incipient insanity was exogenous, and that this was revealed in the 'cerebral excitement and automatic action of the mind', symptoms which had been recorded by De Quincey and Coleridge.[22] In the 1860s and 70s John Bucknill maintained that opium had a central role to play in alleviating insanity, yet Norman Kerr thought it was becoming too fashionable and was undoubtedly a potentially dangerous, destructive, disease-forming drug. By the 1880s George Beard had defined addiction as a symptom of Neurasthenia, one of the many nervous disorders brought on by the strains of progress and modern life. Other physicians, such as Harrington Sainsbury, diagnosed '*habitués*' as suffering from an endogenous condition, a 'moral insanity' born out of the distorted pathology of degenerate stock.[23]

Proponents of the different medical specialisms pronounced on the condition and put forward their various conflicting theories and treatments, unsurprisingly concentrating on the physiological symptoms. Romantic language often seeped into nineteenth-century medical works on drug use, as if that literary genre offered the

---

22 *Blackwood's Magazine*, July-December 1855, 78, p.560.

23 H. Sainsbury, *Drugs and the Drug Habit* (1909), p.106.

most explicit description of this form of insanity and scientific language had yet to construct its own way of discussing the phenomenon. Dr Pereira, in his series of articles entitled 'Narcotics We Indulge In', which appeared in *Blackwood's Magazine* in 1853, made extensive use of the confessional writings of De Quincey and Coleridge. These subjective experiences continued to be widely used as case histories because of the continuing dearth of any other authoritative studies. Using the 'Romantic experience', Pereira wrote of the extraordinary 'fascination' and the 'power of seduction' which opium can produce on the new initiate.[24] Professor Johnston's pragmatically informative and compendious *Chemistry of Common Life* (1855) used the most lyrical prose to conjure up an imaginative empathy with the sensations of taking opium. The opium-eater experienced, he wrote, 'a luxury of sensation … which, even when it deepens (as it sometimes does) into visionary horrors or the wailing phantasmagoria of sorrow', could still be exhilarating if uncontrollable. Much of the work reads, in the professor's own words, like 'excerpts from a Rosicrucian romance'.[25]

But how to explain the link between insanity and addiction? Jones's opinion, that an individual taking opium will experience an involuntarily reaction, accorded with a long theoretical tradition which linked a lack of self-control with mental illness. Porter has argued that 'moralists, medical men and preachers alike could agree that the archetype of madness was the overthrow of mind by carnal appetite', and that he 'who falls passion's slave wilfully, culpably plunges into madness or animality'.[26] Addiction was, *a priori*, one such self-destructive plunge and the symptoms of mania and melancholy had long been seen to bear indisputable similarities to the experiences of those who indulged in opium:

> their Phantasies or Imaginations are perpetually busied with a storm of impetuous thoughts … their notions or conceptions are either incongruous, or represented to them under a false or erroneous image … to their Delirium is most often joyned Audaciousness.[27]

Paradoxically this perceived symbiosis was made manifest with the treatment of insanity with opiates. As early as 1628 Daniel Oxenbridge was employing 'Laudanum Paracelsi' to treat a Mrs Miller, aged 24, 'a Cloth-worker's wife ... mad for two Years, tho' she took many Remedies'. Prefiguring the nineteenth-century debate over mechanical versus medicinal restraint, Thomas Willis recommended in the 1670s that, alongside 'punishments', 'a course of Physick ought to be instituted ... which may suppress or cast down Elation of the Corporeal Soul', and he suggested

24 J. Pereira, 'Narcotics We Indulge In', *Blackwood's Magazine*, July-December 1853, 74, pp.605-28.

25 'Professor Johnston's Last Work', *Blackwood's Magazine*, July-December 1855, 78, p.560.

26 R. Porter, *Mind-Forg'd Manacles*, pp.42-3.

27 Ibid., p.46, quote from Thomas Willis, *Practice of Physic* (1684), p.201.

opiates as efficacious drugs 'frequently noted among all the famous Empiricks'.[28] Blackmore, discussing in some detail the efficacious use of 'pacifick Medicines' in insanity, for the 'disquieting and restless Passions' and for 'Sadness, Dejection, and Fear', believed that opium was 'of singular Advantage in these cases in several Respects:'

> First, as it calms and soothes the Disorders and Perturbations of the animal Spirits; which when lulled and charmed by this soporiferous Drug, cease their Tumults, and settle into a State of Tranquillity: Wonderful it is, how soon the Hurry and Tempest in the Nerves is composed by the Solicitation and Intervention of this prevailing Medicine.[29]

As marvellous as he believed opium to be, Blackmore had reiterated his recommendations for 'limitations' on dosage to avoid any 'ill Consequences', but he stated unequivocally that he had never observed any problems of habit 'where there was no Touch of Lunacy'.[30]

There had always been doubts about the efficacy of prescribing opium too freely. George Young, in his *Treatise on Opium* (1753), was still more circumspect than Blackmore, and he regarded the use of opium 'in hysterics and nervous disorders' as unnecessary and tantamount to giving 'pills to purge folly'. He did, however, alter his opinion with degree and thought its effects dramatic upon those suffering from true 'mania and melancholy', because of its soporific and calming qualities. William Battie declared, in his *Treatise on Madness* (1758), that 'Opium, notwithstanding what hath been before said concerning the great relief obtained by this powerful drug ... is no more a specific in Madness than it is in the Small Pox. For no good whatever can be expected but from its narcotic virtue, and much harm may arise therefrom when improperly administered.' In 1791 Joseph Brandreth stated that 'large doses of opium, in certain cases of insanity, has been ... frequently administered ... with wonderful good effects ... the largest dose I have given ... was like a miracle. From the greatest possible furore, in a few hours my patient was calm and rational'. By the mid-nineteenth century the queen's physician, Sir George Johnson, writing in the *Medical Times and Gazette*, proclaimed that opium might be beneficial 'even before mental disease has actually developed', so that a 'perverted emotion' might be 'held at bay' for as long as necessary.[31] Sir John Bucknill, co-editor with D. H. Tuke of *A Manual of Psychological Medicine* (1858), believed that those who condemned the use of opium in cases of insanity 'had not learned to discriminate the conditions of mental disease in which [the drug] becomes a true balm to the wounded spirit', and he emphasised its central role in the 'whole range of psychological medicine'. Even though controversy reigned, opium remained popular for all nervous conditions,

---

28 R. Hunter and I. Macalpine, eds, *Three Hundred Years of Psychiatry 1535-1860* (1982), pp.122, 191-2.

29 Blackmore, *Treatise of the Spleen*, pp.83-9.

30 Ibid.

31 Hunter and Macalpine, *Three Hundred Years*, pp.395-6.

for it was understood to stimulate the nerves when administered in small doses for depressive states, and to sedate if taken in larger quantities.[32]

In his research on the mid-nineteenth-century Ticehurst House Asylum papers, the psychiatrist Trevor Turner concluded that although a wide range of drugs were used as a regular part of the treatments there, their use was cautious. As a result of the contemporary debates, and coherent with a philosophy based on high staff levels and structured physical and moral care, therapeutic use of opiates was guarded but not condemned or done away with.[33] Whilst it must be recognised that Ticehurst House was a private and philanthropic establishment for the wealthy insane, and therefore a singular institution, the casebooks do provide an insight into attitudes towards the uses of opiates in this and similar environments.

The casebooks give details of the 'exciting causes' of madness in the patients and the physiological effects of the opiates given to them to mitigate their symptoms. A Miss Davies, 'admitted October 31st 1845, age 77', had spent four years in a delusional state, 'chiefly with regard to electricity'. Despite taking a 'composing draught at night' her condition did not abate, and in December of that year she was given 'about 4 grains of Dover's Powder' at nights which seemed to calm her and 'caused her to sleep better than usual, [and] she states that she does not suffer so much from her delusions'.[34] The apparently blanket, or perhaps non-specific, use of opiates for different cases is further highlighted by the treatment of a Miss Fausseth who was admitted on 23 July 1850, age 67, 'labouring under various delusions, imagining her pillow to be filled with snakes, &c. [and] subject to headaches, & sleeplessness'. She was treated with regular 'doses of opium to promote sleep'. A similar treatment was prescribed for an unnamed woman of twenty-nine, an attempted suicide who was 'labouring under delusions of a melancholy kind, fancying her husband and child to be dead'.[35] Opium was the chief sedative remedy for the disturbed and disorientated, but, still, it was argued that the use of narcotics as a curative treatment was a sophistry: opium merely deadened the sick and the real object was to secure quiet wards.[36]

The influential physician and campaigner, Norman Kerr, in his work *Inebriety: A Disease Allied to Insanity* (1884), argued that addiction was a disease and that opium was a cause of insanity rather than a cure. He defined disease in a broad and all encompassing way as 'a condition of the body or brain accompanied by alteration of structure [and] revealed by symptoms [so that] there are the phenomena, natural, mental, moral, and spiritual, due to the operation of this agency'. Believing that 'the intelligent and scientific observer of the origin and development of inebriety can have little doubt of the diseased condition of the inebriate', it was obvious to him

---

32 Porter, *Mind-Forg'd Manacles*, p.185.

33 T. Turner, *A Diagnostic Analysis of the Casebooks of Ticehurst House Asylum 1845-1890* (1991), pp.99, 213.

34 Ibid., p.42.

35 Western MSS, MS 6361-6363, Ticehurst House Asylum casebooks, pp.34, 36.

36 J.M. Granville, *The Care and Cure of the Insane* (1877), p.59.

that these observations applied particularly to opium, which was rapidly becoming a 'fashionable intoxicant'.[37] Addiction in these terms had become a disease whose 'nearest ally is insanity'; indeed, Kerr thought that the aetiology of both conditions was 'in many particulars practically identical', and that there was a 'remarkable likeness in the progress of both'.[38] He explained that an 'exaltation or derangement of the nervous faculties' rendered the insane person or addict unable, 'in some parts, though not necessarily all', to use his reason, control his actions, and more specifically, to exert his will.

The concept of the will in medical theory bridged the gap between the physiological and the psychological and allowed a link between neurology and psychiatry. It described a 'force' for orderly and rational behaviour beyond the pragmatic operation of brain tissue and nervous system, and it provided a focus for therapies and a motivational cause for patients.[39] As J.S. Mill had written, following a period of depression, 'what is really inspiriting and enobling … is the conviction that we have real power over the formation of our own character; that our will, by influencing some of our circumstances, can modify our future habits'.[40] If the will could be educated or strengthened then a greater good might come of it; if, however, it was neglected or given to decay then a moral insanity, voluntary or involuntary, was the price that had to be paid.[41]

Many physicians, including Kerr, believed that because addiction and insanity had been interlinked, it was the duty of the Christian, the philanthropist, and the state to establish homes for the treatment of inebriates in the same way that asylums had been erected for the insane.[42] Kerr understood the addict to be recognisable only 'by the skilled and intelligent physician', and that it rendered the sufferer 'needy' and 'unable to contribute to [his] own maintenance and support'.[43] A Select Committee on the control and management of 'habitual drunkards' in 1872 numbered Lunacy Commissioners as witnesses amongst its members. They found that 'twenty percent of insanity' occurred where 'individuals obey only an overwhelming craving for stimulants to which everything is sacrificed' and where 'self-control is suspended or annihilated; moral obligations are disregarded; the decencies and the duties of private

37 N. Kerr, *Inebriety: A Disease Allied to Insanity* (1884), pp.3-4.

38 Ibid., pp.5-9.

39 Oppenheim, *Shattered Nerves*, p.296.

40 J.S. Mill, *Autobiography* (1873), p.169.

41 Oppenheim, *Shattered Nerves*, p.297.

42 Kerr's speech was printed in pamphlet form and contained a prominent advertisement for the Dalrymple Home for Inebriates, Rickmansworth. This institution was founded in 1884, and licensed under the Inebriates Acts of 1879-99 for the clinical study and treatment of inebriety. It was 'highly approved' by everyone from the *British Medical Journal* to the *Church of England Temperance Chronicle* and the *Sanitary Record*. Kerr was listed as an 'Honorary Consulting Physician'.

43 Berridge and Edwards, 'Special Issue: The Society for the Study of Addiction 1884-1988', *British Journal of Addiction*, 85, 1990, p.991.

life are alike set at nought'.[44] A Dr Robertson, witness to the Select Committee on Lunacy Law in May 1877, gave it as his opinion that the use of narcotic remedies within lunatic asylums was an invaluable and incomparable treatment. But when asked whether he thought such habitual use would have a deleterious effect, he laid the by now familiar stress on judicious medical control of the drug, otherwise, he agreed, it might be as 'prejudicial as the use of any narcotic habitually indulged in'.[45] Addiction, then, rested on who used the drug, how and why it was used, and on the interpretations of the observer: their professional, political, or ethical bent. By the 1870s and 80s the medical journals and national press were referring to 'inebriates', a term which by now included opium users, as 'helpless victims of a vice which they have lost the power to withstand'. They had become parasites, a collective 'burden' and a 'scourge', and were being emotively, if not politically, diagnosed as 'mentally diseased persons hitherto dangerous and often irreclaimable'. A form of guardianship was eventually provided under Section 116 of the 1890 Lunacy Act, to protect addicts from themselves, and the public from them.[46] The conclusions and actions of the committees had definite moral implications, taking the perceived problem of addiction out of the realms of the medical and therapeutic and into the wider social and political spheres.

According to Szasz, in his article 'The Ethics of Addiction', the question of the ethics of collectivism and individualism remains today in society's response to addiction. He argues that 'we can choose to maximise the sphere of action of the state at the expense of the individual, or of the individual at the expense of the state'.[47] In other words, we can support the view that the state has the right and the duty to regulate the life of an individual in the best interests of the group, or we can argue that individual liberty is paramount and that it is the duty of the state to promote and protect it. He sees addiction as a personal choice and, quoting J.S. Mill, from *On Liberty* (1859), argues that it should be left as such unless it causes harm to others:

> The only purpose for which power can be rightfully exercised over any member of a civilized community, against his will, is to prevent harm to others. His own good, either physical or moral, is not a sufficient warrant … In the part [of his conduct] which merely concerns himself, his independence is, of right, absolute. Over himself, over his own body and mind, the individual is sovereign.[48]

Ambiguity held sway: this was a disease *and* a vice. Moral values were attached to it; it was a 'disease of the will' and a 'moral weakness' at one and the same time. When Kerr gave the Presidential address to the inaugural meeting of the Society for the

---

44 R.M. MacLeod, 'The Edge of Hope: Social Policy and Chronic Alcoholism 1870-1900', *Journal of the History of Medicine and Allied Sciences*, 1967, 22, pp.215-45.

45 IUP Select Committee Report on Lunacy Law, p.306.

46 MacLeod, 'The Edge of Hope', pp.225-6.

47 T. Szasz, 'The Ethics of Addiction', in Coomber, *Drugs and Drug Use*, pp.373-82.

48 Ibid.

Study and Cure of Inebriety (SSI) on 25 April 1884, he asked the assembly whether inebriety was 'a sin, a vice, a crime, or a disease'? His evasive, rhetorical reply was that 'it is sometimes all four, but oftener a disease than anything else, and even when anything else, generally a disease as well'.[49] Yet Hill Gibson, speaking on 'Inebriety and Volition' to a subsequent meeting of the same society in the same year, argued that the condition was definitely 'not a physical disease, but a moral vice'.[50] Kerr believed that within the vast and seething mass of the diseased, particularly amongst women, there had actually been a marked and alarming increase in addiction, with the added damage that the 'learned' behaviour of future mothers would intensely affect the 'sobriety of succeeding generations, by stamping an inebriate taint on their progeny'. The disease was thought 'for the most part [to be] the issue of certain physical conditions, an offspring of material parentage, the natural product of a depraved, debilitated, or defective nervous organisation'. It was, he maintained, an inherited tendency, still a diseased state, but one which could be transmitted generationally.[51]

The increasing emphasis on the role of heredity was one of the main perceived symptomatic links between addiction and insanity. The question of heredity influenced many other areas of social concern during the second half of the nineteenth century, and is revealed, for example, in the works of commentators from Henry Mayhew in the 1850s to Havelock Ellis in the 1890s, who evoked a paternalistic passion for uncovering a 'social pathology'. Addiction was seen as a form of inherited profligacy and a predisposition of insanity, a chain of cause and effect stretching across the generations, a result of the inevitability of evolutionary progress.[52] A physician, writing in 1848 on a perceived increase in 'cases of general insanity [which were] certainly disproportionate to the annual increase in population', had attributed this to the opium habits of the working class mothers he treated in his lying-in hospital.[53] And Harrington Sainsbury had been in broad agreement with Kerr when he stated that if there was a fault to be found it would lie 'not with [the drug] but with us'.[54]

Addiction as a disease was embodied in the character of the individual and manifested itself through the will, which, in this instance presented itself as a physiological aspect. The condition could be 'apparently acquired', but it was the quality of the nervous tissue, its stability or instability, which was all important in the resistance offered to temptation, and 'clearly', Sainsbury wrote, 'heredity comes in here'. He praised the 'teaching of biology by means of illustrative types ... strongly

---

49 N. Kerr, *Inaugural Address to the Society for the Study and Cure of Inebriety*, 25 April 1884, p.25. Kerr was at one time a chairman of the British Medical Association's Inebriates Legislation Committee, Medical Officer for Marylebone, London, and a prominent Temperance reformer.

50 Berridge and Edwards, *Opium*, p.155.

51 Kerr, *Inaugural Address*, pp.6, 15.

52 D. Pick, *Faces of Degeneration: A European Disorder, c.1848-c.1918* (1989), pp.195, 208. Scull, *The Most Solitary of Afflictions*, p.238.

53 *Times*, 21 January 1848, p.7, col.e.

54 Sainsbury, *Drugs*, p.60.

advocated by Professor Huxley, amongst others', and, he thought, 'there is little doubt of its wisdom'.[55] It was important, he believed, to recognise that 'while opium relieves pain [it] unfortunately also stimulates, excites, and may bring about a most delightful state of euphoria', and that the question of personal 'moral responsibility', if not 'moral insanity', was paramount and needed to be addressed.[56] Thus the idea of addiction as emanating from an inherent defect was explained and reinforced.

It could be argued that Sainsbury, who, according to *Munk's Roll*, was a self-effacing, deeply religious man with Anglo-Catholic leanings, had applied the belief in original sin to his experiences and observations in the children's hospitals where he practised and assimilated them into his views on heredity, disease, and degeneracy. He believed that it had been 'established that the unborn child may acquire the [drug] habit from the mother', that 'the saturation of the parental system ... must involve a saturation of the offspring', and that 'no more striking object lesson on heredity ... could be given'. The addicted father was also a link in the chain for he tended

> to beget children whose vitality is from the beginning not only seriously impaired, but specifically biased ... every influence in the body tells in the upbuilding of protoplasm [and] the composite protoplasm of the germ borrows its qualities from every form of protoplasm in the parental organism.

The first essential in the prevention of addiction was 'good parentage, [and] the child about to enter the arena of life must come of a good stock [for] shaping the destinies of the race'. Addiction, then, could be seen as a consequence of observable laws, 'traceable deep down into the nature of things' and might not necessarily, therefore, be inherently 'evil'.[57] The onus had been placed, once more, and emphatically, on the character and quality of the individual and Sainsbury was able to dismiss the pressing 'question of accountability' for addiction on the part of the medical profession. In fact, following accusations that the increase in addiction arose from the unfettered distribution of opiates and syringes by physicians, Sainsbury posited that it was 'unquestionably' not evil if it was acquired iatrogenically, that is, caused by physicians themselves through their own therapies.

Medical responsibility and culpability

An extensive account of iatrogenic addiction appeared, significantly, in the *Journal of Mental Science* in 1889. It took the form of a long and detailed letter sent to her physician by a 'Young Lady Laudanum-Drinker' and was described by the editor, in what had by this time become a conventional trope, as her 'Confessions'.[58] She

---

55 Ibid., pp.xi, 214, 223.

56 Ibid., pp.124, 195.

57 Ibid., pp.206, 231-2, 256.

58 'Confessions of a Young Lady Laudanum-Drinker. Dose, Four Ounces Daily, in Two-ounce Doses', *Journal of Mental Science*, January 1889, 34, pp.545-50.

declared that her chief reason for writing was to beg her physician to make known to all, by every means in his power, what a terrible thing 'opium-eating' was. There was no doubt in her mind that the responsibility for her addiction, and for that of many others, lay in the hands of the medical profession. She had tried 'a hundred times to stop it, but never succeeded', and had at last reached the stage at which she didn't 'care a rap' what became of her, 'all the reasoning and affection expended ... being a mere waste of time and love'. She argued that opium was too powerful a drug to expect most people to be able to resist it and she accused the medical profession of complacency and lack of foresight; if they knew 'all the harm those drugs do, as well as the "victims" of them' then why did they do 'precious little to prevent it'? Why did they not advocate 'prevention as well as cure'? Physicians, after all, had it in their power to 'warn those who take laudanum now and then for toothache or a headache, what an insidious thing it is, and how easily they may become the victims of it'. This was how the young woman had begun and 'see what it came to'. The subject needed to be taken seriously and, making a plea for education and information, she argued that if it 'were to be taken up instead of some [subjects] so often spoken of in the health lectures which are now given, it might do some practical good'.[59]

Her diatribe did not go unheeded by the profession, and the same journal carried a reply from W.S. Playfair who wrote 'On the Cure of the Morphia and Alcoholic Habit'.[60] In the cautious view of this physician the 'management of these difficult and unfortunate cases' was 'very unsettled' and, in recounting some of his own experiences treating similar patients, he hoped to facilitate a 'more rational and common sense method than has hitherto been adopted'. Playfair's prescription was not, as had been recommended to the 'Young Lady', an immediate and absolute cessation of her opium, but a 'systematic treatment by complete rest and isolation, accompanied by massage and over-feeding'. He maintained that he had never presided over a failure and that the important thing was to take any means to 'lessen the physical and moral tortures ... which the writer so vividly describes'. Responsibility did not rest solely with the medical profession, he believed, because, in his experience, 'by the time medical advice is sought, there has generally been a complete breakdown, both physical and moral. The patient has neither the strength of mind or will to resist the temptation to which she has succumbed', and indeed, all the cases Playfair went on to provide were of female addicts whose will and nervous systems were generally accepted as being less resilient than her male counterpart's.[61] Henry Maudsley's hypothesis, published in 1874, and accepted without comment by the majority of his professional contemporaries, was that this was 'a matter of physiology, not a matter of sentiment [it is] the energy and power of endurance of the nerve-force which drives the intellectual and muscular machinery'.[62] The female

59 Ibid., p.550.

60 W.S. Playfair, 'On the Cure of the Morphia and Alcoholic Habit', *Journal of Mental Science*, July 1889, 35, pp.179-84.

61 Oppenheim, *Shattered Nerves*, pp.181-232.

62 Ibid., p.190.

state dictated the susceptibility of a woman's nerves, her 'irritability', and her feeble will. Where she combined these traits with addiction she necessarily presented her physician with an almost insoluble problem.

Playfair believed that such cases were 'very difficult and unfortunate', as the female addict laboured under specific 'neurotic conditions'. Indeed, the medical attendant himself also laboured, but under the 'grave responsibility' of refusing to allow narcotics to be placed 'at the uncontrolled disposal of a neurotic woman' who just could not resist temptation. The 'Young Lady' in question, neurotic or not, was incensed at what she saw as the medical profession's lack of interest and action in the consequences of their prescribing opiates and, whilst Playfair admitted some professional responsibility, it was usually, as he believed, a biologically innate secrecy and neuroses that led to female addiction. Women under Playfair's care typically, he believed, had no one to 'control' them, had suffered a 'severe mental shock' or, perhaps, had never recovered from childbirth. They often 'resorted to every practical deviance' to secure their drug, 'sparing themselves no humiliation to obtain it' and 'no reliance could be placed on any statement [they] made'.[63]

Nonetheless, Playfair did accept that some of the blame lay with some of his colleagues, especially if they had allowed an apparently neurotic woman to have free access to narcotics and to drug paraphernalia. He was sorry to say that he had seen 'not one, but many cases directly traceable to errors of judgement of this kind', and still more reprehensibly, he had come across more than one instance in which a colleague had 'actually taught a patient the use of the hypodermic needle, and placed in her hands a bottle of morphia solution to use at her own discretion'. Even so, he suggested tentatively, it might only 'be remarked in passing' that 'the use of the hypodermic syringe is apparently becoming a very common method of taking morphia'.[64]

This tentative response revealed the ambivalence within the medical profession about addiction, particularly iatrogenic addiction. Seymour Sharkey, for example, writing in 1887, suggested that it might all rest on the pressing and ever-present questions of terminology and categorisation. Descriptive archaisms, such as 'enslavement', remained in use but were rapidly losing any innocence they might have had: they were imbued with a linguistic and imaginative potential which could be converted by use and time into concrete fact. 'From time to time', he wrote, 'the English language has been enriched by the addition of words representing varieties of vice, or morbid tendencies', such as dipsomania and kleptomania, and 'now we find ourselves face to face with a new vice ... an uncontrollable craving for morphia'.[65] These sentiments were still being echoed as late as 1909 by Harrington Sainsbury when he hesitantly suggested that it was 'largely a question of terminology and

---

63 'Confessions of a Young Lady Laudanum-Drinker', *Journal of Mental Science*, p.547; Playfair, 'On the Cure of the Morphia and Alcohol Habit', pp.179-84.

64 Ibid., p.181.

65 S. Sharkey, 'Morphinomania', *Nineteenth Century*, September 1887, pp.335-42.

definition' and the recognition of peripheral nervous diseases as clinical facts 'will probably be allowed universally, though [their] naming be debated'.[66]

It is a generally accepted argument, however, that the disease entity of addiction was largely created as a medical condition and a social problem by the introduction of the hypodermic syringe into medical practice. This development gave greater urgency to the disquiet over opiates and to the possibility of addiction, and it had created an uncomfortable paradox. From the 1860s onwards the drug could be administered by the patient him or herself far more effectively than ever before, thus raising the spectre of growing numbers of '*habitués*' or 'morphinists' and inflating the argument for the iatrogenically induced disease of addiction.

Doctors Francis Rynd of Dublin, Alexander Wood of Edinburgh, and Charles Hunter of London, all claimed to have made the initial breakthrough, though there was the usual medical controversy as to who was actually the first to use the hypodermic injection successfully.[67] Rynd claimed he had used the technique in Meath hospital in May 1844, but Wood, apparently unaware of this, published an influential paper on the innovation in 1855, delivered a lecture on it to the British Medical Association in 1858 and subsequently published it in the *British Medical Journal*. Hunter then adopted the method in London, and Howard-Jones, in his article on the development of hypodermic medication, argues that the surgeon, who wrote of the 'tonic effect' it produced 'upon the nervous system', may well have been inducing morphine addiction in his patients during the 1850s. He prescribed its use in cases of 'great mental depression' and also to those 'confirmed opium-eaters' who found that they could take smaller doses subcutaneously than they could by mouth. In 1858 Wood had casually recorded having given over 100 injections to one of his female patients who was suffering from neuralgia.[68] Edward Wilson, writing in the *St. George's Hospital Report* in 1869, gave fulsome, if perhaps sinister, praise to the introduction of the subcutaneous injection of morphia:

> few really important discoveries have glided so silently into every-day use … slowly and surely this new method has won its way and established itself in the profession until there are probably few medical men now to be found who cannot bear testimony, from their own experience, to the marvellous power of narcotics introduced beneath the skin.[69]

But more ominously, and only a year later, T.C. Allbutt, in an article in the *Practitioner*, gave the first warning of the potential problems. 'Among the numerous essays and

66 Sainsbury, *Drugs*, p.106.

67 Berridge and Edwards, *Opium*, p.139; Walton, Beeson, and Bodley Scott, *Oxford Companion*, pp.6-17; N. Howard-Jones, 'A Critical Study of the Origins and Early Development of Hypodermic Medication', *Journal of the History of Medicine*, Spring 1947, pp.201-46.

68 Howard-Jones, 'A Critical Study', pp.209, 214, 230, 232.

69 E. Wilson, 'Notes on the subcutaneous injection of morphia', *St. George's Hospital Report*, 1869, 4, p.19, quoted in Parssinen and Kerner, 'Development of the disease model of drug addiction in Britain, 1870-1926', *Medical History*, 1980, 24, pp.275-96.

records concerning the hypodermic use of morphia which have been published of late', he wrote:

> I cannot call to mind one in which its possible dangers have been considered ... while my fears were indefinite, I felt the time had not come for me to speak. Now my experience has been greater, I have a large number of cases before me, and yet the uncomfortable fear of mischief is growing rather than diminishing.[70]

He had seen hypodermic morphia used in cases of neuralgia for periods of months and years, and yet these people seemed as 'far from cure as they ever were' except that they were all finding relief in the 'incessant use of the syringe' believing that, without it 'life would be insupportable'. Allbutt asked whether morphia was encouraging the very pains it was intended to relieve, or:

> if not, does it at any rate induce in those who use it constantly, an artificial state which makes its further use a necessity? Are the subjects of morphia injection, that is, liable to become depressed, relaxed, irritable and dependent on a new habit of constant intoxication? If this be so, we are incurring a grave risk in bidding people to inject whenever they need it, and in telling them that morphia can have no ill effects upon them so long as it brings with it tranquillity and wellbeing.[71]

In 1871 F.E. Anstie expressed his worry that the practice had become a 'comparatively common household remedy among certain classes of society for some years past'. He thought it was used mainly by women who injected themselves, or had their servants do it for them, whenever they had an attack of 'nervous depression and sleeplessness.[72] A decade later Dr Westland wrote to the *British Medical Journal* detailing his observations in cases of 'habitual administration of morphia in large quantities by hypodermic injection'. His conclusion was merely that he had never met any 'persons who were more miserable themselves, and a greater source of discomfort to their friends'.[73] Oscar Jennings published many such case-histories including one of a lawyer aged 35, who was addicted to morphia for ten years after having been 'taught the practice by his medical attendant'. His physician seemed to have been 'certainly culpable, having propagated the use of the syringe amongst his patients in the most imprudent manner'.[74] The argument for iatrogenic addiction was not a popular one amongst the medical profession and it has been suggested that patient's constant demands for morphine and oft-repeated injections were sufficiently lucrative to cause many physicians to turn a blind eye.[75] Certainly,

---

70 T.C. Allbutt, 'On the Abuse of Hypodermic Injections of Morphia', *Practitioner*, 1870, 5, pp.329-30.

71 Ibid.

72 Howard-Jones, 'A Critical Study', p.233.

73 *British Medical Journal*, 2 July 1881, vol.2, pp.30-1.

74 O. Jennings, *On the Cure of the Morphia Habit* (1890), p.88.

75 Howard-Jones, 'A Critical Study', p.233.

as D.H. Tuke wrote in 1882, 'hypodermic injections of morphia ... have had their strenuous advocates during late years'.[76]

As Berridge has pointed out, it seems that, despite this evidence, and a widespread belief in the predominance of the female opium addict, there is little material to support the reported extensive use of self-administration of the hypodermic syringe. She suggests instead that any problem of 'excessive' use of morphine was in fact largely confined to members of the medical profession, causing this aspect of opium-taking to be artificially emphasised.

Opium addiction within the profession was not a new phenomenon: as early as 1807 Thomas Trotter, commenting on the dangers of falling victim to a habit, wrote that 'there is reason to believe, that even medical men themselves, have of late, entered into the indiscriminate use of opium'.[77] And in 1853, when Dr Pereira's articles on 'The Narcotics We Indulge In' had appeared in *Blackwood's Magazine*, it had seemed necessary to include a disclaimer assuring readers that the author was not himself an opium-eater.[78]

J. B. Mattison, a physician writing in the *Medical Record* in 1883, and believing that the 'subtly ensnaring power of opium is simply incredible to one who has not had personal observation or experience', recorded that he had recently dismissed six 'medical gentlemen' from his care.[79] To the best of his knowledge they had all recovered from their morphia addictions. Such were the numbers and such was the problem, that he had felt driven to write on the subject which he assumed must 'be of personal and painful interest' to many of his professional readers. To verify his claims of addiction amongst his peers he quoted other physicians who estimated, variously, that a third of their patients were medical men and that they formed a much larger proportion compared with any other professional class. One authority wrote that, in his opinion, 'quite an incredible number of our colleagues have fallen victims to it, and many have only just escaped'. Moreover, and more damning, he declared that:

> if medical men are charged; and it is to be feared, justly, with the propagation of this disease, owing to their carelessly, or for mere convenience sake, leaving morphia and a subcutaneous syringe with the patient, it may be regarded as their punishment that the demon morphinism finds among them his favourite victims.[80]

Mattison dismissed the idea that his claims and concerns were in any way 'alarmist'. The reality was that the 'anxious hours, the weary days, and wakeful nights, such

---

76 D.H. Tuke, *History of the Insane* (1882), p.485, quoted in Scull, *Museums of Madness*, p.170.

77 Trotter, *Nervous Temperament*, p.137.

78 *Blackwood's Magazine*, July-December 1853, 74, p.628. Hayter also felt the need to include such a disclaimer, *Opium and the Romantic Imagination*.

79 J.B. Mattison, 'Opium Addiction Among Medical Men', *Medical Record*, 9 June 1883, 23, pp.621-3.

80 Ibid.

as the experience of every busy practitioner so often involves' were reason enough to drive them to the 'peculiar power that opium possesses'. Every physician was subject to 'inroads on his mental health and physical well-being, expos[ing] him more than any other to the various influences which stand as factors in the etiology of this disease'. That addiction was a disease was now an undoubted medical fact to Mattison, and many of his colleagues were succumbing and suffering from it. He speculated that the proportionally large numbers of addicted physicians seeking help could be explained by the 'secretive character of this disorder': simply, they would refuse to entrust their health to charlatans in order to preserve their anonymity as a lay-person might do. Rather, they would eschew the 'specious promises [and] beguiling blandishments' and 'extend their confidence to those whose skill and experience' would 'secure the aid which scientific treatments can now surely afford'.[81]

Even as Mattison claimed the disease of addiction as medicine's own he was aware of the dangers of its prevalence amongst its servants. 'This very knowledge and the frequent employment of this potent agent for evil as well as good' could breed familiarity and diminish any 'fear of its ill-effects, and make easy the occasional taking … which so soon forges the fetters of confirmed addiction'. And neither were medical men immune to the new neurotic disorders that it was thought could often lead to the chronic misuse of opium. 'Any physician afflicted with neurotic disease of marked severity', he wrote, 'and who has in his possession a hypodermic syringe … is bound to become, sooner or later, if he tampers at all with the potent and fascinating alleviative, an opium *habitué*'. Whilst proclaiming medicine's progressive 'scientific treatments', the profession needed, at the same time, to warn against its parallel pitfalls.[82]

According to the physician Oscar Jennings, one medical man in four was a 'drug *habitué*', most usually a 'morphinist'. Based on cases discussed in his works on addiction, published over a twenty-year period from 1890, he estimated the proportion of medical addicts to the total of cases to be as high as ninety per cent.[83] He was appalled at the indifference and even hostility of the medical profession to this situation, declaring it 'notorious', particularly when, in his estimation, one-fifth of mortality amongst his colleagues was caused by addiction to morphine. His critics considered it to be 'a waste of time to study the subject, or to try to help those who do not intend to help themselves', and that 'the best attitude towards such patients was to have nothing to do with them'. One eminent physician had remarked derisively that Jennings might 'as well ask us to cure the habit of lying, or the habit of stealing, as that of … opium. He, and many others, believed that, disease or no, the 'moral obliquity of mankind does not come within the range of *materia medica*'.[84] Jennings profoundly disagreed; he had himself been addicted to morphine for twenty-five

81 Ibid.

82 Ibid.

83 Jennings, *The Morphia Habit and its Voluntary Renunciation (A personal relation of a suppression after twenty-five years' addiction). With notes and additional cases* (1909).

84 Ibid., *The Morphia Habit*, pp.v-viii.

years and believed that this experience provided him with particular insights into the condition and its treatments.

The introduction to his first book on the subject in 1890 verged on the apologetic as he self-deprecatingly wrote in his 'Little Work' that people might find his suggestions tiresomely and 'disagreeably exacting'.[85] By the time he published his last major study in 1909 he had, as it were, come out, and the title bravely said it all: *The Morphia Habit and its Voluntary Renunciation (A personal relation of a suppression after twenty-five years' addiction)*. His work became contentiously well known and his estimates of 'medical addicts' were, unsurprisingly, attacked in print by some of his enraged colleagues for the perceived slur on the profession. As Jennings had commented, 'it has been decided by the profession at large that morphine *habitués* are invariably cheats and liars, degraded beings unworthy of confidence', and he was himself being tarred with the same brush.[86]

Nonetheless, Jennings's theories on the treatment of addiction, if not his opinions, were well received in the journals. The *Lancet* 'heartily recommended' them to those who desired to relieve their patients of the 'thraldom of this terrible habit'. The *Medical and Surgical Review* considered that his 'therapeutic discoveries [had] laid an important branch of suffering humanity under a deep debt of gratitude'; the *Hospital* thought the works 'should be read by every practitioner in charge of a morphia subject'; and the *British Medical Journal* saw him as 'the recognised authority thereon'.[87] Professional rivalry in this new therapeutic field could be fierce, and Jennings himself, when not complaining that his ideas were being used and passed off as their own by other less scrupulous doctors, had 'no hesitation in declaring that before this there was no rational treatment of the morphia craving ... at all'.[88]

Jennings felt that his contemporaries did not or would not really understand addiction, and he thought their 'so-called' methods of treatment were 'brutal, barbarous & inhuman'. The most common methods consisted only of suppressing the use of the drug 'slowly or semi-brusquely', and, according to him, they would always lead to an eventual relapse due to 'ignorance, or rather, indifference, concerning the means of alleviating the craving'. The real question was one of 'attenuating and rendering bearable the craving', for Jennings perceived and measured addiction by the levels of distress experienced in the withdrawal process. He had his own precise and certain conception of the nature of the morphia 'craving' and drew up a rational 'Analysis of Craving' to show that it had component parts which could be treated systematically. According to this detailed scheme most addicts suffered from a 'condition of ordinary ennui' and the want of mental stimulation could be felt as a 'craving-yearning'. Translating this into physiological terms, he described it as a

85 Ibid., *On the Cure of the Morphia Habit* (1890), p.vii.

86 Ibid.

87 Ibid.

88 Ibid., pp.47-8; *On the Cure of the Morphia Habit Without Suffering* (1901), pp.1, 4.

'want of molecular change in certain cerebral centres' which could then be intensified into a distress, or an 'ento-peripheral' pain, that resulted from 'the representation of a future in which such cravings will never be satisfied'. Addiction was then present as every subsequent recurrence of the sensation would be heightened by auto-suggestion of the means of satisfaction, and by the 'abeyance of ... the will ... into fixed yearning for the accustomed stimulant'. If every 'morbid sensation' during the addict's past had been treated with opium, then every malaise in the future would, by association, suggest the idea of craving.[89]

In Jennings's experience the addict was always profoundly discouraged by the certainty that, once the craving came on, he or she knew that they would suffer increasing distress until the opium was obtained, and that that would then become their only goal. His treatment therefore consisted of: motion, whether in a hammock or through massage; sufficient time; a slow reduction of dose; and, crucially, the re-education of the will. Order and regularity were paramount to the cure, and in this the regime echoed the traditional humoural theory of maintaining health and well-being. Jennings believed that addicts also fell prey to a 'mania of injecting': that the morbid, sordid pleasure derived from the act of injecting something under the skin held as great a fascination as the effects of the morphia. It was important then to remove this pleasure and to allow only rectal injections, which he thought, on the whole, would probably be a less attractive temptation.[90] This, and the necessity of a change of environment to remove a patient from their 'perverted associates' and from their ability to 'tyrannise' their families, prefigures the twentieth-century theory of set and setting as indicative of this behaviour. But it also isolated the addict, declared him or her a patient, placed in a form of quarantine, and in danger of metaphorically infecting, or being infected by, others.

Acknowledging that medical knowledge and ideology are in constant flux, Shorter, in his work *From Paralysis to Fatigue: A History of Psychosomatic Illness in the Modern Era* (1992), has proposed the possibility that patients continually change the manifestations of their psychological anxieties to accord unconsciously with the reigning medical paradigms of the day. Shorter argues that the display of myriad symptoms, especially nervous ones, results from complex codes of illness behaviour subtly indicated by physicians and internalised unconsciously by the patients.[91] In a similar vein Jennings believed that his task was complicated because his patients were capable of fabricating their responses 'in order not to hurt the feelings' of their doctor.

In his case histories he also discussed his use of placebos and, occasionally, trickery which produced the results that both he and his patient expected.[92] A female

89 Ibid.

90 Ibid., *On the Cure of the Morphia Habit*, pp.16, 30, 48, 74; *On the Cure of the Morphia Habit Without Suffering*, pp.14, 30-40, 51, 53, 63.

91 Shorter, 'Paralysis: The Rise and Fall of a "Hysterical Symptom"', *Journal of Social History*, Summer 1986, 19, pp.549-82; Shorter, *From Paralysis to Fatigue*, chapter 1.

92 Jennings, *On the Cure of the Morphia Habit Without Suffering*, pp.22, 174-7.

patient in her fifties but, in his estimation, with the appearance of a seventy-year-old, 'manifested all kinds of hysterical symptoms, and claimed to be suffering from the most acute craving'. Despite his generally empathetic and liberal attitudes to *habitués* and their claims, Jennings was decidedly sceptical in this case for here, he thought, was an irrational and puerile woman unable, because of her sex, to exert her will or her intelligence. What his account shows is that she exerted her will but not in the direction required by her doctor, thereby behaving, according to him, in a quite irrational way. What she had asked for was an element of control over her own treatment, to the extent that she herself would judge the progression of the reduction of her doses of morphine, and that Jennings should oversee and 'countersign' it. She had, he remarked in self-exoneration, been treated by '*dozens*' of other doctors, 'some of them of the very highest eminence', who had abandoned her case as soon as she had 'set herself to seriously harass them'. Jennings circumvented her wishes entirely by deceiving her with a placebo, allowing her to think 'all the time that she was working her own sweet will'. One evening, deciding he would not lend himself to her 'nonsense any longer', tired as he was of 'carrying on the comedy of a scene each night before I would allow myself to give the (imaginary) extra morphine', he revealed his deception. He was apparently amazed at her reaction. Instead of the gratitude he had expected she again exhibited the 'strange perversity of the hysterical temperament' and became audaciously enraged at his treatment of her, persuading her husband to take her home. She died six weeks later of an overdose.[93] Her doctor had denied her any self-control, had denied her any strength of will by virtue of her physiology, even though he believed that 'the whole treatment of the morphia habit turns upon a proper comprehension of the psychology of *habitués*'. Unfortunately this was a psychology already based upon prejudice.[94]

Jennings sometimes described his gentleman *habitués* as difficult but, as often as not, his female patients were hysterical. One young woman, addicted to both cocaine and morphine, had been referred to Jennings by her husband, a medical man and morphine *habitué* himself. She had enlisted the assistance of a 'flighty' maid whom she allowed to stay out half the night in return for a supply of drugs entered into household expenses as meat and groceries, and 'speculating on her mistress' passion, the servant had already made her pay with jewellery - that very day bracelets which she had pawned for over £50'. Jennings illustrated what he saw as the hopeless perfidy of his female addicts by revealing that when this patient was within 'a fraction of a grain of complete suppression' she had bribed the wife of a chemist to send her morphia in a double-bottomed *bon-bon* box at the price of two pounds a gramme; the cost price being about three pence'.[95]

The women invariably displayed, the doctor recorded, 'every hysterical symptom imaginable' if not 'violent excitement ... at not being able to have [their] own way'. A young woman of twenty-eight, whose case notes he published in 1901, received

93 Ibid., pp.175-6.

94 Jennings, *The Morphia Habit*, p. 291.

95 Jennings, *On the Cure of the Morphia Habit*, (1890), p.76.

his admonitions and recommendations with 'speechless indignation' and 'tearful reproaches', apparently following up this 'hysterical' reaction ten minutes later by 'gaily talking about some absorbing matter – toilette, jewellery or the races'.[96] Taking her responses at face value Jennings encapsulated common assumptions about women and applied them to his understanding of aetiology and to his diagnosis and treatment of them.

Diseases and drugs had long been presumed to act differently on women and men. According to humoral theory women were inherently cold and moist and men warm and dry, and, according to Aristotelian theory, women were irrational and emotional whilst men had command of reason and logical analysis. In the mid-nineteenth century Thomas Laycock, in his work *A Treatise on the Nervous Diseases of Women* (1840), had stated that 'woman, as compared with man, is of the nervous temperament ... more easily acted upon by all impressions', and her presumed subservience to man was given contemporary credence by the evolutionary theories of Darwin and Spencer. These reinforced traditional beliefs influenced gender attitudes to addiction as with any other condition, particularly, though, in this case when the alleged weakness of the female will informed virtually all medical models of women's nerves, health and character.

The nervous prostration suffered by these women was considered pathological and related to the biological female state, where the reproductive life of women was understood as a form of ill-health. Woman was a helpless victim of her physiology, denied the same recourse to personal choice and responsibility which was afforded to her male counterpart.[97]

That the addicts advised and treated by Jennings were well-to-do is not in doubt; these were educated people, higher degenerates, whose condition could be indulged. They had the requisite time and money, and were to be 'credited with good faith and encouraged ... instead of being suspected of a desire to relapse'. It was unwise to put moral pressure on them as this 'class of cases' already had the required sensitivity and only needed guidance for their 'dormant will', and, of course, to be 'desirous of giving up the habit'.[98] Jennings believed them to be essentially creatures of impulse, often hysterics, and prey to their desires. It was always the patient who was '*the chief complication in his own case*', and any addict who relapsed did so 'because it is his pleasure'. Paul Rodet, commenting on Jennings's work in 1897, remarked on the way he had 'characterised this psychosomatic state in calling it at once a sensation and a sentiment. It gives the sensation of an unappeased appetite and of an unsatisfied desire'.[99] Thus he reiterated the tension and the struggle to understand the relationship between the physiological and the psychological as it was manifested in addiction.

---

96 Jennings, *On the Cure of the Morphia Habit* (1901), pp. 172-3.

97 Oppenheim, *Shattered Nerves*, pp.181-2.

98 Jennings, *On the Cure of the Morphia Habit Without Suffering*, pp.154-5.

99 Ibid., pp.95, 118, 119.

Having struggled to define the perceived new disease and to realise the numbers who were now discovered to be suffering from it, the medical profession was forced to address itself to the wider implications. The classification of the condition as a nervous disease and a form of insanity had gained currency in medical circles from the late eighteenth century, and, from the mid-nineteenth century onwards the inclusion of the opiate user alongside the 'habitual drunkard' as someone legitimately requiring treatment gained most credibility. Professor Alfred Taylor, giving evidence to the Select Committee on the Sale of Poisons Bill in 1857, had put forward the opinion that chronic opium users might receive a certificate every six months to ensure their supply from a druggist for that period. This suggested that physicians accepted the belief that addiction was a disease, that addicts were sick, that they needed their drug and that they should be given it. It also affirmed the argument of the medical profession that physicians should be able to practise their science as they saw fit, emphasising their professional struggle and innate paternalism. Taylor's idea of a maintenance dose was reaffirmed in one of the central recommendations of the Rolleston Committee on Morphine and Heroin Addiction in 1926.[100] It still carries weight as one of several theories of addiction in currency today.

Concluding remarks

It is apparent that the medical profession found it difficult to agree on the specifics of addiction; nor were they always certain that it actually existed. Further, their often conservative and self-conscious pronouncements were seen to carry not only a practical, but also, by a form of emotional and intellectual extrapolation, a heavy moral weight. This was, with few exceptions, a moral pathology built upon an Augean swamp of presupposition. And, try as some of them might, they could not divorce addictive behaviour seen as a pathological symptom from the same seen as a way of life, even if a wilfully degraded or an enfeebled and degenerate one. Addiction came to be understood not only as a slavish condition, but also as a false way of being and so necessarily against nature. It was anti-social and self-absorbed, unproductive and therefore decadent. It was based on internalised energy with no appreciable functional good and was therefore destructive, both for the individual and for society. The assumed unhealthy and shameful privacy of the self required remedy through the intrusive explorations of the medical profession. And, this being the case, where whole areas of feeling and reason were ignored, then the nineteenth-century medical concept of addiction as a disease was reductive and impoverished. Physicians had attempted to define, and so, consciously or not, to possess and order the inner life of the imagination, the secret and private self, and they were unable to resist prescribing moral judgements along with their empirical understanding of pharmacodynamics. This was a case, it sometimes seemed, of the unimaginative in pursuit of the unattainable. Significantly, and as early as 1807, Thomas Trotter had

100 G. Edwards, 'Opium and After', *Lancet*, 16 February 1980, pp.351-4.

bleakly and prophetically remarked that 'a methodical history' of diseases, including narcotic addiction, was 'almost impossible'.[101]

101 Trotter, *Treatise*, p.166.

Chapter Seven

Late Nineteenth-Century Theories of Addiction: The Pathologist, the Physician, and the Philosopher

The swing of the pendulum

> It is to be remembered that a bodily infirmity is not the only thing to be corrected ... the soul itself has received impressions that are incompatible with its reasoning powers. The subject, in all respects, requires great delicacy and address; and you must beware how you inveigh against the propensity; for the cravings of appetite for the poisonous draught are to the intemperate … as much as the inclinations of nature for a time, as a draught of cold water to a traveller panting with thirst in a desart (sic). Much vigilance will often be required in watching these cravings; for they are sometimes attended with modes of deceptions, and a degree of cunning, not to be equalled.[1]

The sensitivity and insight apparent in the above paragraph, written in 1804, belies the common assumption that, because of their relative lack of scientific knowledge, early commentators and theorists on addiction had only the crudest understanding of the condition as it is understood today. To illustrate this misconception we can look at another work, published in 1986, which argues that 'the idea that alcoholism … is a disease has been growing in popularity for the last 20 or 30 years, and would now be regarded as a mark of liberal and enlightened opinion'.[2] We can see in these two studies, written nearly two hundred years apart, something of the perpetuity of theories of addiction as they have been elucidated over the past two centuries. They reveal the unchanging nature of the debate's raw material, by which is meant the addictive state, and the constantly changing social and medical constructs that surround it.

The former piece, written by the physician Thomas Trotter, discusses the idea of 'received impressions on the soul' whilst Heather and Robertson, authors of the latter, describe addiction as learned behaviour dependent on 'crucial social and psychological determinants' as well as being a physiological response or 'resonance'.[3] Addiction itself emerges as a constant and, perhaps, a natural state: it is the individual

---

1 Trotter, *Essay on Drunkenness* (1804), p.172.

2 N. Heather and I. Robertson, 'Is Alcoholism a Disease?', in Coomber, *Drugs and Drug Use*, p.38.

3 Ibid.

drug user, the cultural environment in which a drug is experienced, and the language that has been variously used to describe it, that provides the apparent deviations.

Up to the mid-nineteenth century most discussion of habitual drug use concentrated on the symptoms and consequences rather than on the aetiology of the perceived problem. Some of these apparent effects had quite definite moral intentions and connotations, partly because they were thought to unleash other varieties of unwanted, inconvenient human desire. A Dr Thompson, writing in the *Medical Times* in 1840, stated that in his opinion opium used purely as a stimulant was never a medicine and, further, it 'acted as an aphrodisiac and subverted all morality' affecting, particularly, 'all that was good and virtuous in women'.[4] Suppression of the 'luxurious' use of opium was, in this sense, a behavioural rather than a pharmacological or physiological question; unless, and until, morality was thought of in pathological terms.

The early nineteenth-century scientific interest in the effects of habitual use, scant as it was, was due primarily to the work of the new breed of toxicologist. In 1850 Christison noted in the *Lancet* that, although 'opium intemperance ... had notoriously become a somewhat prevalent vice, both among the working classes and in the wealthier ranks of society in this country', very little had yet been added to medical knowledge of its effects since his own earlier works on poisons in the 1820s and 1830s.[5] And, importantly, little had been added to the knowledge of the causes of this addiction. Many theories had been produced on matters of longevity, on the various miseries and discomforts consequent on the habit, and on remedies for those who had overdosed themselves, but few, if any, had appeared that addressed the question of the root of the compulsion itself.

Where such works existed they relied on an uncomfortable but eminently powerful combination of pathology and morality. As an example of this a medical article on addiction, in this instance to alcohol, published in 1850, unabashedly included ideas attributed to Archdeacon Jeffreys of Bombay. In his sermon the cleric had stated that, out of all the magnificent gifts of Providence and 'all the enjoyments of life ... there is not one of them which the wickedness of man does not more or less abuse'. Jeffreys lambasted the evils of excess in general, invited and sustained the idea of disease as divine punishment, and used the Aristotelian metaphor of the body politic brought down by a parasitic corruption. These arguments gave a traditional credibility and force to his words and he emphasised the heuristic injunction that:

> if it is to be found by experience that there is something so ensnaring in the article itself, or something so peculiarly untoward connected with the use of it in the present age, that the whole amount of crime, and misery, and wretchedness connected with abuse of it greatly

4 *Medical Times*, 1840, 1, pp.162-3.

5 Christison, 'Supplement to the preceding Paper on the Habitual Use of Opium, more especially the Mode of Cure', *Lancet*, 1850, 1, pp.531-8.

exceeds the whole amount of benefit arising from the right use of it; then ... it becomes the duty of every good man to get rid of it.[6]

It was not until the 1860s that discussion of addiction began to make a concerted move towards a systematic application of an emotionally colder, more candid empiricism. There was a valiant and deliberate attempt to eschew the moral overtones which, though influential, did nothing to advance a purely objective understanding of addiction which was already being designated a disease entity. This more positivist approach, born of the process of medical professionalisation and specialisation, would assure the creation of a scientific model of addiction but, ideally, the task would require the application of unbiased practitioners. The incorporation of information and ideas into a coherent scheme had to pass muster within the scientific community as a whole in order that it should be accepted as a valid and respectable scientific theory. But this process alone, whilst it invited an exchange of comment and discussion, could not help but hinder impartiality.

The question of the possibility of labouring fiercely to establish what might not even actually be there, i.e. a *disease* of addiction, was answered by the self-confidence of scientism. Arguing for the pre-eminence of empirical methodology, John Stuart Mill, in his *System of Logic* (1872), stated explicitly that 'it is a law that there is a law for everything'. He believed that what science ideally aimed for was 'a set of laws giving necessary and sufficient conditions' for all events. And a cause would always be the result of the conjunction of several conditions, that is, 'in general, there will be a plurality of causes' to be considered.[7] That associations occur under certain conditions had been recognised since Aristotle clearly stated this law in his treatise *On Memory*.[8] These specific associations are understood as '*habits* or *patterns*'; they are not general and are themselves conditional upon certain other things having happened. Still, in the 1990s, the idea that the mutable concept of addiction can only be understood in a multi-disciplinary way is illustrated by the following statement issued by the European Collaborating Centres in Addiction Studies, and it reveals the constancy of this fundamental argument over time:

The field of addictive behaviour encompasses many disciplines in biomedical and socio-behavioural fields – principally pharmacology, biochemistry, neurophysiology, endocrinology, psychology and sociology. Clinical scientists also need an understanding of psychopathology, natural history, treatment evaluation and other psychological variants.[9]

6 W.B. Carpenter, *On the Use and Abuse of Alcoholic Liquors, in Health and Disease* (1850), pp.xv-xvi.

7 J.S. Mill, *System of Logic* (1872), bk iii, chapter v, para.6.

8 V.G. Hardcastle, 'What We Don't Know About Brains', *Studies in History and Philosophy of Biological and Biomedical Sciences,* March 1999, 30, pp.99-100.

9 Report from European Collaborating Centres in Addiction Studies (1995).

This chapter explores the construction of the hypothesis of addiction as it was approached by three prominent and influential theorists in the second half of the nineteenth century, the pathologist F.E. Anstie, the physician George Beard, and the philosopher Herbert Spencer. These men were major proponents of the formal, paradigmatic knowledge about the concept of addiction as it gained scientific acceptance. The pathologist's taxonomy of drugs and drug reactions, the physician's construction of a disease, and the philosopher's theories of psychology all embraced and elucidated the concept of addiction.

The Pathologist

F.E. Anstie (1833-74) was an eminent and influential physician whose works became standard texts for the medical profession during the late nineteenth century. Beginning as Resident Physician-Accoucheur and Anaesthetist at King's College Hospital, London in 1859, he thereafter held a series of distinguished medical appointments in the capital.[10] A radical and philanthropical man, he was an advocate of medicine as a career for women, helping to found the London Medical School for Women, and he sat on the committee investigating the administration of London's Poor Law Infirmaries which led to improvements in poor-law medical relief. For several years he was on the editorial staff of the *Lancet* and in 1869 became sole editor of the *Practitioner* after acting as joint editor in the first year of that journal's existence.[11] Anstie's dynamic, professional and altruistic career, and his dedication to furtherance of medical knowledge was beyond reproach.

One of Anstie's major taxonomic works, *Stimulants and Narcotics: Their Mutual Relations* (1864), provided a definitive outline of the actions of drugs, including any addictive properties they might have. This study was intended to clarify therapeutic classification in 'the light of recent clinical observation and physiological experiment'.[12] As a physician he was greatly exercised by the opacity that had distinguished mid-nineteenth-century ideas on the actions of drugs and this could be remedied, he believed, only with the growth of objective empirical knowledge. Anstie recognised that he had undertaken a task of immense difficulty in attempting both to ascertain and differentiate the hurtful effects of drugs from the useful, and to clarify an apparent discrimination between what was a food and what a poison. In order that he might reach a truly empirical and unambiguous conclusion he assured his readers that his analysis would necessarily exclude the 'special moral and religious aspects' which he saw already accompanied the question. He did not deny these aspects existed but he believed that they required a firm basis in fact so that empirical science would not be obscured. He would not, for example, argue against the use of a drug just because some individuals might wish to abuse it: he thought

10 Anstie was appointed Physician at Chelsea Dispensary and Assistant Physician and Lecturer on Forensic Medicine at Westminster Hospital in 1860, becoming Physician at Westminster in 1873. He was also Physician to Belgrave Hospital for Children and Consulting Physician to the Royal South London Opthalmic Hospital.

11 *Munk's Roll*, p.144.

12 F.E. Anstie, *Stimulants and Narcotics: Their Mutual Relations* (1864), pp.1-20.

that both the medical profession and the general public should be provided with a systematic treatise on the broad and important facts as to the daily use of narcotics and stimulants. Further, he argued that the everyday use of these substances was not an 'out-growth of modern corruption' as some commentators insisted it was. Anstie wanted to approach his subject without the distorting effects of preconceived assumptions or a judgemental position.

If such a laudable analysis could be achieved the medical profession might then arrive at a positive understanding, tangible and capable of physical demonstration, and free from any perversion, which, he thought, 'in human hands [it] is liable to'. On the contrary, he maintained that the common use of drugs was validated by the sanction of immemorial custom and that there was 'no period of history, as there [was] absolutely no nation upon earth' in which one could not find evidence of this behaviour. It was a 'practical fact', he insisted, that nations, let alone individuals, could not, and never had been able to do without narcotics. To support this, the reader's attention was drawn to the acknowledged authority of Professor Johnstone's 'ingenious' map in his *Chemistry of Common Life* (1855). This work revealed that little of the earth's surface was without any indigenous narcotic plant, and that these were freely indulged in by 'native peoples', 'not merely for medicinal purposes, but for everyday use'. Anstie further forcefully conveyed his argument with the following:

> Coffee-leaves are taken, in the form of infusion, by two millions of the world's inhabitants. Paraguay tea is taken by ten millions. Coca by as many. Chicory, either pure or mixed with coffee, by forty millions. Cacao, either as chocolate, or in some other form, by fifty millions. Haschisch is eaten and smoked by 300 millions. Opium by 400 millions. Chinese tea is drunk by 500 millions. Finally, all the known nations of the world are addicted to the use of tobacco, chiefly in the form of smoke; otherwise, by snuffing or chewing.[13]

As has been noted elsewhere in this book, substances that an early twenty-first-century observer might not automatically class together, such as coffee and opium, are here given apparent parity. Extrapolation of this argument means that it is not the particular substance which carries damaging potential but the individual who responds idiosyncratically to the 'special powers' of a drug according to his or her 'temperament'. This theory was considered in chapter five and can be attributed to adherence to the traditional principle of humoural individualism. Recent definitions of drug addiction take the element of potential into consideration too, so that an addict is seen as someone vulnerable to the compulsive heavy consumption of drugs with 'abuse potential'. In order of risk of addiction, cocaine and amphetamines have greater abuse potential than opiates and nicotine, which in turn have greater addiction potential than alcohol and related drugs, which are greater than cannabis, hallucinogens and caffeine.[14] Whilst Anstie was eventually to arrive at what appears to be a traditional theory of drug action based on the user's idiosyncratic type, he

13 Ibid.

14 Segen, *Current Medical Talk*, p.12.

nonetheless shied away from the older language of subjection to vital forces and humoural balance. He was ready to debunk what he thought of as the source of much fallacious theory which, he maintained, had induced the authors of recent essays on therapeutics to cling to injuriously outmoded and pedantic theories.

Some of these 'virtually dead' notions were based on the premise that certain drugs, when administered in larger than necessary doses, produced poisonous effects which gave the appearance of being merely an exaggerated response to the ordinary medicinal action. He volunteered opium as a good example, in that it promoted sleep in a medicinal dose, but induced coma in a 'poisonous' one. It had been accepted that the latter state was the extreme development of the former; *ergo* the action of opium was essentially the same in all doses. But Anstie argued that there was too wide a discrepancy between the two states and that any physiologist worth his salt would realise that there was considerable doubt as to whether coma was exaggerated sleep at all. So that, where previous dogmatic assertion had held that there were either stimulants or narcotics, both with fixed properties and actions, Anstie was now confident in describing a third, intermediate class possessing the qualities of both.[15] By making a shift in the understanding of drug action he was also paving the way for a change in the understanding of the drug taker.

In elucidating this argument and the question of avoiding moral judgement on everyday drug use or abuse, he turned to examining the actions of particular substances. Holding up common salt as an example, he remarked that in small doses it was a welcome addition to the dinner table, 'a perfectly indispensable article of human food', but still one 'without which we should perish miserably'. In medium doses it remained safe and was indeed, a useful emetic medicine. But in extremely large doses it became an irritant poison and could be responsible for death. So that the action of salt, in the first instance termed 'vital', could alter and become 'morbid'. Similarly with iron, which as a normal element of the blood prevents anaemia, in large doses causes fatal inflammation of the stomach and bowel. Even arsenic, according to the contemporary results of medical practice, could be tolerated and even considered beneficial in small amounts, but if the dose was increased it might prove to be a powerful poison leading rapidly to death.

Evidence relating to the 'dangerous enjoyment' derived from a poisonous arsenic habit was recorded in the *Lancet* in 1852. Users adapted their doses to suit their particular 'constitution', taking the drug to relieve enervation and bolster vigour. But if the arsenic-eater was deprived of his or her supply it was a recognised fact that they would be overtaken with symptoms resembling poisoning. The author described common withdrawal symptoms: the sufferers succumbed to 'a feeling of general discomfort, attended by a perfect indifference to all surrounding persons and things, great personal anxiety, and various distressing sensations arising from the digestive organs ... and especially difficulty of breathing'. In his opinion there was but one remedy, *viz*, 'a return to the *enjoyment* of arsenic'. Concluding his argument

15 Anstie, *Stimulants and Narcotics*, pp.1-20.

the author stated, as an inevitability, that, as with the practice of opium-eating, once the drug habit was commenced it became a necessity.[16]

Anstie argued that there was no defining certainty as to when, or under what particular circumstances, a substance might be a medicine or poison or even a food, so any prejudices against consumption were necessarily based on false or inaccurate premises. To clarify the central uncertainties he needed to reappraise the formal teaching of the day that separated these agents into such rigid categories. He drew attention to the practical experience of medical men, to the application of these categories and terms depending on the conditions under which the substance was administered, and most importantly to the dosages given. The physician, he argued, should resist the strictures of conventional judgements on these drugs, recognise that their properties and actions might produce particular results, but understand that these would be wholly dependent on diverse use. Thus the medical man could not afford, as it were, to infect his analysis with misplaced morality. There was no inevitability about the question of drug use. One man's food might be allowed, under this system, to be another man's poison.

Anstie considered that rational empiricism could be the only response to traditional influences and attitudes that were mere, if convincing, hypotheses. The empiricist must guard against negligently supporting erroneous theories. If a particular substance was found to produce a particular effect, he urged that every care should be taken to discover the precise means of its physiological action in order that fictitious but convenient ideas and explanations might be avoided. Contemporary hypotheses about stimulus and the action of drugs were, according to Anstie, rooted in ideas 'most excellent and useful' *in their day* and adopted 'by ancient philosophers ... for the purpose of helping themselves some little way further towards the comprehension of things which it was impossible ... that they could fully understand'. It seems that Anstie saw himself as treading a similar path of investigation and knowledge but as being further along the journey to understanding and as having to necessarily debunk some earlier conclusions. The ancient physicians had, he thought, so vividly portrayed their ideas that many which were intended to have been interpreted figuratively had instead been understood literally and had lasted into the mid-nineteenth century as fact, as 'fundamental truths in medical belief'. Beliefs, he argued, such as those on stimulation and excitability, unquestionably came out of this accumulative process of 'mutilation and ... encrustation'. If terms such as stimulation and excitability were still to be employed they required new definitions and limitations of their meanings. The new empirical physiology could then effectively replace the traditional idea of an essence, like 'a demon or demons' residing in the nerves, which could be propitiated with cordials, soothed with anodynes, excited with stimulants, or inflamed into action.[17]

Moreover, in order not to alienate his more conservative peers, he argued that this did not dismiss the 'participation of spirit' in the living body in favour of too

16 *Lancet*, 1852, 1, p.85.

17 Anstie, *Stimulants and Narcotics*, pp.64-5

materialistic a view. Indeed, the contrary would hold sway, as the 'true character of mind - changeless, eternal, unconfined to time or space' would be better realised. And, if it was, then expressions constantly used to describe the actions of inebriants, such as 'stimulating the mental powers' or 'reducing the mental excitement', would not treat the intellect as merely some form of 'secretion from the brain' to be acted on by the use of narcotics. The assumption that particular mental states could literally be created or removed would be seen to be 'unfounded and mischievous'. All the medical profession could know was that the brain should ideally be 'placed in that state of nutrition, &c. which represents material health, and ... the best chance has been afforded for the mind to act rightly'.

Present-day science is just as ambivalent about the extent of its knowledge of the brain. An article, 'What We Don't Know About Brains', published in *Studies in History and Philosophy of Biological and Biomedical Sciences* (1999), was intended to serve 'as a serious warning to those who wish to use neurophysiological considerations in bolstering philosophical or psychological arguments': for as the author argues, 'we know not whereof we speak'.[18] The reader is warned that he or she 'will get educated guesswork and piece-meal investigation held together by dogma and faith'. What they will not get are any definitive answers, for 'we do not even know how to tell that we are on the right track in our empirical testing of the brain'. Anstie's own cautious methodology still accords with this 'approach in illustrating the depth of our ignorance in neuroscience'. The twentieth-century author emphasises the need 'to outline the guiding doctrines in ... research and highlight their weaknesses and fundamental points of conflict [for] these doctrines shape how we interpret data – indeed, they determine what we call data in the first place'. There was, and still is, 'deep conflict over what counts as evidence for a claim, over what counts as a good scientific explanation, and over what the fundamental unit of cognition is'.[19] That there has always been more than one fundamental doctrine in any science, and that there continues to be disagreement on the most basic of points leading to paradigm shifts in formal knowledge, tells us something about how much we still do not know.

Anstie maintained that nothing could accurately be known about the effect on the mind of any deviation from an ideal physiological state. Traditional medical treatments of large doses of narcotics such as opium for those suffering, for example, from acute mania or derangement must be seen to have been highly dubious under these terms.[20] And what he refers to as 'the continuous "stimulation" so frequently had recourse to' in chronic illness also presented the nineteenth-century doctor with a problem.[21] The first dose of a stimulant produced, Anstie wrote, the 'highest degree

---

18 Hardcastle, 'What We Don't Know About Brains', pp.69-127.

19 Ibid.

20 Anstie, *Stimulants and Narcotics*, pp.66-7.

21 Ibid., p.76, 'The operation of stimulus upon the organism ... may be classified under six heads, according as they refer to the mind, to sensation, to muscular motion, to secretion, to circulation, or to nutrition'.

of exaltation [before] depression sets in: in order to prevent the development of this state we repeat the stimulant medicine ... presently comes the recoil, which we again immediately arrest by a fresh dose, and so on'.[22] The influence of such agents on the mind he saw as producing an 'exaltation of mental activity that would not be possible without the use of extraordinary means'. Anstie carefully examined these 'mental phenomena' with a view to supporting his claim that they were due to the removal of 'pre-existing obstacles' in the mind rather than to a 'direct instantaneous increase of the mental powers'. He looked at alcohol, hashish and opium, which he regarded as substances being most typical of the 'inebriant medicines'.

Whilst the initial phenomenon of alcoholic intoxication resembled 'excitement', Anstie did not hesitate to acknowledge the contemporary truism that the 'emotional and appetitive part of the mind' was in action, while the intellect, on the contrary, was 'directly enfeebled'. Everyone, he believed, would recognise how the 'lower and more animal nature' obtruded itself in the behaviour of a drunken person, and this in direct proportion to the lessening of his or her intellectual activity and functional capabilities. Accordingly, then, he argued that a drunken, 'violent outbreak of the passions' was due not to any stimulation of the emotions but to the removal of 'the check ordinarily imposed by reason and will'. The influence of hashish, too, was seen to be the result of the removal or 'paralysis' of these checks, or inhibitions, and their release of a 'great exhilaration of spirits, of an unreasoning character [and] the involuntary production of fantastic mental images'.[23]

The influence of opium, however, presented greater difficulties of definition as the mental phenomena caused by its use were, he remarked, much less familiarly known. It was commonly held that in the great majority of European constitutions opium produced no discernible mental excitement, but most Orientals, and perhaps some Europeans whose 'habits of life are peculiar', experienced a condition 'very remarkable, and very difficult to analyse'. These individuals might take large doses of opium without succumbing to stupefaction or death. Indeed, they claimed that their minds seemed to work with greater freedom and that they would experience exhilaration of their spirits. They also, he thought, exhibited a fixed indisposition to hard work of any kind. All these effects might last for eighteen to forty-eight hours following a significant dose, to be succeeded by a heavy, semi-comatose sleep. Anstie, when experimenting with a large dose of the drug upon himself, reported that he felt only 'depression and misery', whilst the effects produced by smaller doses included 'a warm and comfortable feeling ... in the whole body [with] no particular desire for sleep'. He thought it impossible to determine the true meaning of this information without far more precise data. He concluded, however, that the evidence he had collected revealed a 'really poisonous and depressing influence operating upon some portion of the brain simultaneously with the apparent stimulation'. That being the case he believed that any desired medical effect could and should be achieved only

22 Ibid., p.71.

23 Ibid., pp.76-81, 119-21.

with small doses, for the 'use of full narcotic doses [was] both needless, and, in most cases, injurious' in that they could potentially lead to a habit being formed.[24]

Appealing again to common experience Anstie wrote with assurance that 'everyone knows ... that there *is* a fatal necessity for the individual who has once habituated himself to the *narcotic* effects [of a substance] to go on augmenting his daily allowance'.[25] Such excessive habitual use of narcotics, he continued, would lead to a degradation of the nervous centres, partly due to the direct repeated action of the 'poison' but also to the 'small amount of common nutriment taken', particularly so when opium or alcohol were the drugs in question. The 'abnormal nutrition' of the immoderate opium-eater resulted in physical degeneration which might or might not tend to shorten life, but, where death was premature it was, in the majority of cases, due to 'mal-nutrition which has been set up, and not to a special disease of the nervous system' nor to a *disease* of addiction. From this point Anstie posited that it was easy to understand how and why it became more difficult for the *habitué* to induce the same effects as before without increasing the dose of his chosen narcotic. In a creative leap of logic he argued that, as the individual's 'quantity of nervous tissue ... ceased to fill the *rôle* of nervous tissue' by succumbing to the deadening effect of narcotism, there was 'less of impressible matter upon which the narcotic may operate', and hence it was that the confirmed opium-eater required more and more of his 'accustomed narcotic to produce the intoxication which he delights in'. The user must literally have had to saturate his blood with the 'poison' if he were to 'enjoy once more the transition from the realities of life to the dreamland, or the pleasant vacuity of mind, which this or the other form of narcotism has hitherto afforded him'.[26]

Thus Anstie explained his theory of addiction through philosophic and scientific means, relying on his clinical observation and experience and physiological experiment. Ostensibly he believed that to revise ancient but commonly held assumptions about these substances and their effects, both the medical profession and the layman would need to put aside any preconceptions. But, he wrote, nearly every drug known to man constituted a poison in large doses and it was clear to him that 'evil always lies so near the good'. In discussing what he saw as the excessive indulgence in narcotics of some individuals, he had, despite his intentions, manoeuvred himself into addressing that 'interference of moral considerations with our physical problem' which he had promised to avoid in his introductory chapter. At the very least he realised that the moral perspective, though distorting, would not go away.

The 'baser part of narcotic temptation' was to be discovered in the physiological need he had described and in the fact that it required prolonged and determined use to reach such a condition of craving. The 'genuine debauchee of narcotism', he wrote, '*loves to be drunk* with his particular narcotic. He wants nothing more

24 Ibid.
25 Ibid., p.471.
26 Ibid., pp.242-4.

than to be carried away from all the actual surroundings of life, and placed in a fool's Paradise, filled with illusions of sensual delight.' This, Anstie maintained, was quite a different experience to that of the 'unwary' person who took a narcotic in a moderate amount to relieve weariness, but mistakenly believed that by increasing the dose he would increase his relief. Narcotics taken in this manner were better regarded as 'a special variety of foods' in that they provided sustenance for the sick and so reflected the 'wisdom of Divine Providence'. This sick person had no '*desire to be drunk*', and it was this trait that was '*the* secret of the hopelessly downward progress of the ordinary victim of intemperance'. For the debauchee it was not only the physiological process of need which he had set to work; it was firmly rooted in his 'debased moral nature [that] loves the unnatural delights which can only now be obtained by such an increase'. And this moral debasement, according to Anstie's own observations, appeared to him to be more inherent in the individual's character than to be a product of the progressive action of the narcotic 'mischievous as that may be'.[27]

The argument was, then, that there were considerable numbers of people born with distinct hereditary tendencies to 'sensualism', people who had 'peculiar' latent susceptibilities that might be made manifest by narcotic drugs. These individuals he regarded, much as Trotter had done more than half a century earlier, as the 'victims' of narcotic excess, for once they had experienced the 'vividness' and 'force' of their revived emotions and impressions they could not resist the desire for repetition. They became slaves to an inescapable 'vicious sequence', and required increased doses of their drug as their physical degeneration progressed and as the 'devitalizing influence' continued to be exerted. Such a victim could rarely if ever be free of less than a poisonous amount of his narcotic, he could never recover from the damage he had done to his nervous tissues, and so must have constant recourse to his drug or suffer the terrible consequences. The habitual and tormented feelings of 'languor and depression' experienced in the intervals between debauches would be unfavourably contrasted with the delightful sensory and mental delusions created by the narcotic, and the debauchee would be driven to return again and again to his *bête noire*.[28]

The action of the narcotic in excessive doses provided, in Anstie's opinion, a temporary glimpse of the 'original basis of the character' of the drug user rather than an imposed and artificial inspiration to certain deeds or thoughts. He railed against what he saw as misleading and specious speculation on the mystical effects of opium, or 'the narcotic delirium which is sometimes sought for by the literary dilettante', a sentiment that Thomas Huxley might have envisaged when he described 'the great tragedy of Science' as being that of the 'slaying of a beautiful hypothesis by an ugly fact'. Anstie pointedly suggested that the eloquent account of De Quincey's pleasures and pains in the *Confessions* was 'truly a poisoning', but nonetheless he considered it a striking illustration of the remarkable powers

27 Ibid., pp.244-5
28 Ibid., pp.246-8.

of opium.[29] The 'involuntary fancy' conjured up by the drug was, to the doctor's scientific mind, a form of 'mental disturbance' and 'an extraordinary characteristic of most non-congenital forms of insanity'. As such it was merely a pseudo creative response presenting 'unreal *spectra* to the eye, or unreal feelings to the senses'. Anstie explained De Quincey's graphic descriptions of this 'painting, as it were, upon the darkness all sorts of phantoms', and his experience of the distortion of time and spacial perception as being nothing more spiritual than past impressions crowding into the consciousness in a 'pell-mell' fashion, thereby giving the illusion of being creations rather than mere reproductions.[30]

Much of De Quincey's account was, nonetheless, in accordance with conversations Anstie had held with several opium-eaters, and it corresponded closely with the phenomena produced by other narcotics. Anstie himself had experienced an instance of 'involuntary phantasy' after taking a large dose of belladonna. He had swallowed the extract in order to verify or disprove the statements of others on the supposed innocuousness of the drug. On retiring to bed at eleven o'clock he had taken about a grain and a half of good quality belladonna and then awoken at four in the morning in a state of slight delirium. Everywhere he looked around his familiar room there appeared to be swarming legions of the 'most disgusting spectra'. 'Insect creation' was Anstie's own particular horror and he was forced to suffer spectral cockroaches seething and crawling about him and over him for two hours until they began slowly to fade away. His personal experience and clinical observation confirmed him in his belief that different narcotics paralysed the brain in different ways whilst capriciously unveiling latent impressions and emotions. He adamantly denied any suggestion that there was anything creative in this process, 'notwithstanding the opinion of so able an observer as De Quincey'.[31] The doctor perhaps thought it unnecessarily imprudent, or even self-revealing, to record fully De Quincey's view that 'if a man, "whose talk is of oxen," should become an opium-eater, the probability is, that (if he is not too dull to dream at all) - he will dream about oxen', or in this case, cockroaches.[32]

Coleridge had put it thus: 'Doctors are *shallow* animals; having always employed their minds about Body and Gut, they imagine that in the whole system of things there is nothing but Gut and Body'.[33] Anstie had obdurately encapsulated his material system thus:

> Narcosis may be, therefore, understood to be no less than the severance of the copula of life ... The mental disturbances to which the action of narcotics may give rise, are as follows:- Loss of the reasoning faculty, of the moral sense, and of the power of voluntary recollection: prominence of the emotional and appetitive instincts; delirium, involuntary memory, and involuntary fancy; partial or total loss of consciousness ... The disturbances of the sensibility include:- delusive feelings of heat or cold ... formication (creeping

29 Anstie, *Stimulants and Narcotics*, p.149.

30 Ibid., pp.195-7.

31 Ibid., pp.197-9.

32 De Quincey, *Confessions*, p.21.

33 Griggs, *Collected Letters of Samuel Taylor Coleridge*, p.256.

> sensations) ... perversions of the other special senses; actual paralysis of common sensation ... undue slowness, with abnormal feebleness.[34]

Once the victim had crossed Anstie's '*poison-line*', dictated by his individual and idiosyncratic condition, he was vulnerable purely to the physiological actions of the narcotic, however these might affect the mind. Charles Baudelaire, in an essay first published in 1858, described the narcotic experience of hashish as 'a vast dream ... [that] will always preserve the particular tonality of the individual'.[35] He wrote dismissively of the 'lazy man [who] has searched hard in order to introduce artificially the supernatural into his life'. Not only had this dreamer foolishly succumbed to a false paradise; he was 'mastered' by it and 'his misfortune is that this is only ... the already dominant part of himself: *He wanted to be an angel, he has become a beast*'. The essay was written for 'the worldly and the ignorant [all] those eager to experience exceptional delights', in part to show that they would find nothing 'miraculous ... absolutely nothing but an excess of the natural. The brain and the organs ... will show only their ordinary, individual phenomena, enlarged, it is true, in number and energy, but always faithful to their origin'. This poet and this doctor both believed that 'man will not escape the fate of his physical and moral temperament: the [drug] will be, for his familiar impressions and thoughts, an enlarging mirror, but a clear one'.[36] It was understood that the drug user, with his or her particular and specific inherent characteristics, was the catalyst for the hitherto inert, though potentially effective drug. The drug was deemed to be, it could be said, blameless, whilst the user was seen to be innocent or corrupted according to his or her hereditary make up and the manner of drug use.

But clinical empiricism had its detractors amongst some physicians anxious to treat emerging disease entities. It was said that whilst the 'experimenters were swallow[ing] their own experiments', the practitioners were becoming impatient at being 'forced' to wait for them to determine by these means what could be safely indulged in. They were in a professional hurry to pursue the 'best road by which we shall arrive at the truth' and thought that the 'great question of stimulants and narcotics in all its vast relations to hygienic morality, political and social economy, and science in general' should be answered through experience and observation.[37]

The Physician

If an established and empirical scientist such as Anstie found it difficult to separate moral questions from his enquiries, other figures, such as George Beard, found it

---

34 Anstie, *Stimulants and Narcotics*, pp.174-5.

35 Charles Baudelaire, 'On the Artificial Ideal: Hashish' (1858), in Strausbaugh and Blaise, *The Drug User Documents*.

36 Ibid.

37 G.M. Beard, *Stimulants and Narcotics: Medically, Philosophically, and Morally Considered* (1871), pp. 27-8.

impossible if not inconceivable. He was the personification of the physician as moral mechanic. 'Why is it', he asked, 'that man, with his powerful will holding him back from wrong, and his rich and varied moral nature lifting him above the temptations of passion as no other animal is favoured, yet becomes the worst of animals in the presence of opium?'[38] Beard's rhetorical question lay at the centre of his work on *Stimulants and Narcotics: Medically, Philosophically, and Morally Considered* (1871). Though an American physician, Beard's work was accorded considerable attention and achieved validity in England, and his ideas were assimilated into the majority of systematic and clinical volumes published here. Born in 1839 in Connecticut, he was the son of a minister and the grandson of a physician. He was educated at the College of Physicians and Surgeons in New York from which he graduated in 1866, having written his thesis on themes of longevity and the value of work. He kept a diary during his college years that revealed an inner struggle between religion and science, and the possibly consequent bouts of depression, nervousness, and indigestion he suffered. Beard was a member of the New York Medico-Legal Society, a Fellow of the American Academy of Medicine, Vice-President of the American Academy of Medicine, and a member of the American Neurological Association. He had both a private and a dispensary practice, and published widely on the emerging science of neurology that was developing simultaneously in Europe and North America in the late nineteenth century as part of the general trend towards medical specialisation.[39]

Beard's views on the actions of stimulants and narcotics were largely in accordance with Anstie's, but he had none of his colleague's reticence concerning the distorting effects of emotive moralising on the findings of science. In agreement with the accepted thinking on the excessive use of these substances, Beard repeated the argument of the revelation of the true nature, or 'organisation', of an individual when drugged. But he argued that it was a matter of something he imaginatively termed 'moral chemistry', a sort of quasi-scientific catch-all term. He described how, by removing the restraints of society, which existed to repress the 'lower and degrading passions', man could not help but reveal himself 'as he is' rather than as who 'he thinks he should be'.[40] Beard made no bones about his belief in an ideal of 'civilised morality', a socio-religious medical system based on a 'strict discipline of work and sexuality' which naturally and firmly precluded any form of intemperate behaviour.[41] He exhibited the contrast of the new self-confidence and optimism of science with a Christian doctrine espousing the 'fallen', corrupt and broken nature of mankind.

---

38 Ibid., p.70.

39 E.T. Carlson, 'George M. Beard and Neurasthenia', in E. Wallace and L. Pressley, eds, *Essays in the History of Psychiatry* 10th annual supplementary volume to *Psychiatric Forum* (1980).

40 Ibid., pp.116, 122.

41 Carlson, *George M. Beard*, p.56.

Paradoxically he enlisted Coleridge in support of his argument, noting that the poet and inveterate opium user had once remarked that if he lived by the seashore he would preach fifty-two sermons a year against the wreckers.[42] Beard either failed to realise, or he ignored the full context of self-loathing and impotence which prompted the analogy. If Coleridge had actually lived by the sea, he himself was aware that he wouldn't have been able to resist any of the spoils as they were washed up on the beach. Anstie had been particularly wary of laying himself open to confusions such as this and had attempted to avoid moralising as a means, not only of preventing distortion, but also of deflecting exposure to the scathing criticism of medical sceptics.

Beard's mission allowed no such fears. Excessive use of stimulants and narcotics was, according to this doctor, particular to humankind for, in his own great chain of being, whilst the 'lower animals indulge in other passions more recklessly and grossly than man', no one had ever heard 'of a cow, or a horse, or a sheep, or dog, or cat, or a hog, going down to a drunkard's grave'. He did note, however, that monkeys had been known to get drunk and that Darwin had said that these close cousins of man also, on occasion, smoked tobacco with undeniable pleasure. These vacuous and specious arguments, directed at the emotions, sit in a peculiar juxtaposition with Beard's professed 'scientific reasoning', though it is true that he did intend his work to be appreciated 'in a manner at once scientific & Popular'. He may perhaps have thought it worthwhile to sacrifice some professional credibility amongst his peers so that he might get across to the lay person his campaigning polemic against the various and ingenious manifestations of intemperance that so exercised him.

Beard proclaimed, in his self-important and often overblown fashion, that he himself 'would rather risk [his] own life by jumping off Niagara Falls, than by forming the habit of opium-eating'.[43] He did, however, record trying a large dose of hemp so that he could better compare its effects on the nervous system with other substances such as opium, which, presumably, he had also explored with self-administration. This experiment he settled to his satisfaction but also for a while, he recorded, to his utter terror as he had been unable fully to control his mind and was fearfully conscious of the fact. He had felt 'strange indescribable feelings' in his head and the ability to summon up a single coherent sentence had escaped him completely. He vowed he would never forget this 'night of horror', during which he had believed himself to be 'in the midst of a great amphitheatre, the seats of which were filled with little devils', all of whom were incessantly bowing to him and grinning maniacally at his agony.[44] Beard had experienced nothing approaching the promised 'visions of heaven' that others had assured him were there for the taking. Having indulged in narcotics purely to further scientific knowledge he was evidently pleased to note that such pleasures were probably felt by only a very few,

42 Beard, *Stimulants and Narcotics*, p.70.

43 Ibid., p.149.

44 Ibid., pp.64-6.

and he considered himself a sufficiently evolved and civilised being to be beyond a condition of slavery to any of these substances.

The problem of intemperance weighed heavily on Beard and his investigation was a search for the 'truth' about stimulants and narcotics and their use that had, he maintained, 'greatly extended and multiplied with the progress of civilisation ... especially in modern times'.[45] The question, he wrote, in true Gradgrind fashion, was 'pre-eminently one of fact'. The emotions, 'powerful and indispensable' though they were, would not determine the answers unaided, no matter how fervently he wished they could. But neither could the chemical and physiological trials of scientists assist, for these, in his opinion, were still in their infancy and, as the 'experimenters swallow[ed] their own experiments', the results were less than valid. He considered trials on 'lower animals' to be ineffective as well, as all creatures so far 'summoned to the witness stand and required to give their opinion concerning the effects of these substances ... have pretty unanimously and very emphatically expressed themselves in opposition to ... the stimulating and narcotizing substances that are so popular with their human brethren'. No, Beard argued that the 'one and only way' to discern the truth was 'by *experience*, by trying them on large numbers of individuals, and observing their effects over a long period of time'.[46]

The doctor was not alone in his overweening ideas. Benjamin Ward Richardson, in his work *Diseases of Modern Life* (1876), thought it 'doubtful whether the freedom of the subject ought to be permitted to extend to the uncontrolled self-indulgence in these poisons', arguing that 'indulgence in narcotics ... is an entire departure from natural law' and that it indicated an 'unsound reason which requires to be governed by sound reason'.[47] Beard did not suggest that his notional programme of experiment and control should be carried out involuntarily, but he was no real friend of the individual, especially if he or she were of that section of society he termed 'the poor, and ignorant, and idle classes that have almost always been found among highly civilised people'. These lesser mortals were, in his opinion, exposed to the same stimulants and narcotics that 'the civilised brain-working orders' had devised and employed, yet they lacked sufficient 'moral force and elevation to use [them] with decorum'. As such, he argued that they could not but help fall into the habit of using them to enormous and detrimental excess.[48] And any continued use of the drugs was far worse in women than in men because, he believed, the 'more nervous the organisation, the greater the susceptibility' to habit. But, contrarily, if she was a woman of the 'intellectual and refined classes', the opposite appeared to hold true, and her finer organisation would naturally be repelled by such base things. Oddly, this was not because her moral force was any the greater, but because her temptations

45 Ibid., p.24.

46 Ibid., pp.26-30.

47 B.W. Richardson, *Diseases of Modern Life* (1876), pp.495-6.

48 Beard, *Stimulants and Narcotics*, p.38.

were fewer. In the pursuit of a profitable disease even virtue was interpreted in the negative.[49]

Where Beard perceived addiction to be the result of vice he posited the idea of a 'vicious organisation [of an] entirely healthy brain ... and surroundings' as the cause. This type he found most frequently 'among the ignorant and degraded, and among the so-called criminal classes'. But vice itself could also be understood as a disease, and then it was most commonly manifested among the 'intellectual and cultivated' whose greater sensibility would preclude a wilful descent into viciousness. However addiction presented itself, Beard saw it as a question of the inescapable nature of things, almost as a form or a result of original sin. Amongst the 'degenerate', he thought it arose from an hereditary deficiency where the brain was not 'modelled after the type of good men, but rather of bad men, and it is as natural for them to get drunk, or to stupefy themselves with opium or tobacco, as it is for other and better formed natures to study philosophy, to write poetry, to succour the destitute, or to fall on their knees in prayer'. Under this system the addict and the philosopher could almost never be one and the same, but both would always act 'in obedience to organisation, for which they deserve but little praise or blame'.[50]

Despite his protestations about whether they deserved blame or not, addicts undoubtedly received their due from Beard, who made his less than scientific gut feeling clear when he stated, for example, that the degenerate 'loves ugliness for its own sake' whilst the cultivated is merely a victim of a consequential elevated sensitivity. Unfortunately for the better class of sufferer an excess of sensitivity could lead to addictive behaviour, but the only way out of it was to raise one's moral tone still higher, thus risking a greater fall. Beard's moralising had caused him to fence himself in with yet another contradiction. In this case the cure was itself the disease.

For the highly sensitive and often diseased Beard had a special place in his pathological scheme. He became known as the father of 'Neurasthenia', a disease entity that included the symptom of susceptibility to the drug habit, and he promoted and elucidated it in a manner bordering on the entrepreneurial. All discomforts, ailments and dissatisfactions, great or small, could be brought under its socially coveted title, including the uncontrollable desire for stimulants and narcotics.

A neurasthenic might suffer from any one, or a combination, of an exhaustive list of symptoms provided by Beard. These were, he wrote, 'familiar to all medical men yet usually under different names', and the disease was 'liable to attack all functions and organs'. Diagnosis, not surprisingly, was 'oftentimes extremely difficult' and 'absolutely impossible' without close scrutiny of the individual patient.[51] This was a fastidious condition, acutely suited and delicately tailored to a particular medical market at a particular time. Tom Lutz has argued, in his recent anecdotal history

49 Ibid., pp.51, 116-17.

50 Ibid., pp.72-3.

51 G. Beard, *A Practical Treatise on Nervous Exhaustion (Neurasthenia), its Symptoms, Nature, Sequences, Treatment* (1880), pp.11-12, 90.

of nervousness, that the disease was a medical metaphor for perceived economic, social, and even cosmic decay: the excessive stimuli of modern life taking its toll on unprepared humanity.[52] Gosling, in his work *Before Freud*, describes it as being the inevitable price Victorians saw themselves as paying for the march of progress and civilisation, whilst Carlson, in his article 'George M. Beard and Neurasthenia', sees it as analogous with the contemporary law of the conservation of energy.[53] Carlson argues that Beard was influenced by the work of his friend Thomas Edison, and that he merely applied the idea of a dimmed electrical current to the weakening of the human nervous system. In searching for a diagnosis for such a draining of the vital life-force the physician and the patient could look to a myriad indications that included the following:

> Tenderness of the Scalp.- Cerebral Irritation.- Dilated Pupils.- Sick Headache and Various Forms of Head Pain.- Pain, Pressure, and Heaviness in the Head.- Changes in the Expression of the Eye.- Congestion of the Conjunctiva.- Disturbances of the Nerves of Special Sense.- Neurasthenic Asthenopia.- *Muscoe Volitantes*.- Noises in the Ears.- Atonic Voice.- Deficient Mental Control.- Mental Irritability.- Hopelessness.- Morbid Fears.- Astraphobia or Fear of Lightening.- Topophobia or Fear of Places.- Agoraphobia or Fear of Open Places.- Claustrophobia or Fear of Closed Places.- Anthrophobia or Fear of Society.- Monophobia or Fear of Being Alone.- Phobophobia or Fear of Fears.- Mysophobia or Fear of Contamination.- Pantaphobia or Fear of Everything.- Flushing and Fidgetiness.- Frequent Blushing.- Sleeplessness.- Bad Dreams.- Insomnia.- Drowsiness.- Tenderness of the Teeth and Gums.- Nervous Dyspepsia (*Dyspepsie Asthénique*).- Deficient Thirst and Capacity for Assimilating Fluids.- Desire for Stimulants and Narcotics.- Dryness of the Skin.- Abnormalities of the Secretions.- Abnormal Dryness of the Skin, Joints, Mucous Membranes.- Sweating Hands and Feet with Redness (PalmarHyperidorosis).- Salivation.- Tenderness of the Spine (Spinal Irritation) and of the whole Body (General Hyperaesthesia).- Cocyodynia.- Peculiarities of Pain in the Back.- Heaviness of the Loin and Limbs.- Shooting Pains simulating those of Ataxy.- Podalgia (Pain in the Feet).- Tremulous and Variable Pulse and Palpitation of the Heart (Irritable Heart).- Local Spasms of Muscles (Tremors).- Dysphagia (Difficulty of Swallowing).- Convulsive Movements, especially on going to Sleep.- Cramps.- Special Idiosyncrasies in regard to Food, Medicine, and external Irritants.- Sensitiveness to Weather.- Sensitiveness to Cold or Hot Water.- Sensitiveness to Changes in the Weather.- Sunstroke brings on many Symptoms of Neurasthenia.- Localised Peripheral Numbness and Hyperaesthesia.- A Feeling of Profound Exhaustion Unaccompanied by Positive Pain.- Ticklishness.- Vague Pains and Flying Neuralgias.- General or Local Itching (Pruritis).- General and Local Chills and Flashes of Heat.- Cold Feet and Hands.- Nervous Chills.- Sudden giving way of General or Special Functions.- Temporary Paralysis.- Diseases of Men (Involuntary Emissions, Partial or Complete, Impotence, Irritability of the Prostatic Urethra).- Diseases of Women.- Oxalates, Urates, Phosphates, and Spermatozoa in the Urine.- Gaping and

---

52 T. Lutz, *American Nervousness, 1903: An Anecdotal History* (1991), pp.xii, 3.

53 F.G. Gosling, *Before Freud: Neurasthenia and the American Medical Community, 1870-1910* (1987) p.10; Carlson, *George M. Beard*, p.53.

Yawning.- Appearance of Youth.- Rapid Decay and Irregularities of the Teeth.- Hemi-neurasthenia.[54]

Perhaps unsurprisingly, Beard was not without his critics. Sir A. Clark, Physician to the London Hospital, regarded this list as 'an assemblage of incoherent indications ... borrowed more or less freely from inchoate forms of insanity, and from almost every disease of the nervous system'. Emphasising Beard's inherent contradictions he pointed out that, for the most part, sufferers were 'always excitable and sometimes depressed ... procrastinating, fragmentary, and inconstant', yet there were 'nevertheless, to be found among them the greatest workers of the times ... fastidious, refined, and cultivated, they fall occasionally under the dominion of sensuousness and the lower emotions'. Clark thought the term neurasthenia to be 'unscientific, inaccurate, and misleading', though he was forced to admit that it had won general acceptance within the medical profession. In the face of 'a just but feeble opposition' he grudgingly admitted that it was 'to be found heading a chapter in almost every one of our systematic and clinical works'.[55]

Addiction was an unavoidable condition of the true neurasthenic. Beard argued that, should the nervous system lose its force under the barrage of discomforts he described, 'it leans on the nearest and most convenient artificial support that is capable of temporarily propping up the enfeebled frame'. A drug, such as opium, that could provide the desired 'ease, sedation [and] oblivion', might be resorted to at first in an isolated incident but it would finally, and inevitably, become a devastating habit. He believed this 'tendency' to be a latent and hereditary one which would not become apparent until some affliction or distress robbed the brain of its nervous force. Men, and particularly women, might 'resort to the drug-shop' not merely for the relief of pain but also to gain respite from an 'exhaustion, deeper and more distressing'.[56] These victims of chronic exhaustion then, through no fault of their own, were tempted to treat their 'depression [and] hopelessness' with ever increasing doses until they became addicted, until they had had succumbed to 'Opio-Mania'. The 'servant became the master - the patient the slave', and in some dire cases 'two poisons, alcohol or opium' were taken together in excess.

It was Beard's opinion that 'the evil of opium-taking in nervous exhaustion' was a growing one and he was being 'constantly called upon to treat patients who have added the morphine habit to their weaknesses and pains'.[57] But due, perhaps, to the paucity of the pharmacopoeia, he often found himself forced to treat the opio-maniac with opium itself. It was, he thought, 'excellent for many phases of neurasthenia', but he was always wary for he had been 'obliged to treat too many cases of the opium habit' to be too reckless in his dispensing.[58] He thought that physicians, whom

54 Beard, *A Practical Treatise on Nervous Exhaustion*, p.xvii.

55 Sir A. Clark, 'Some Observations concerning what is called Neurasthenia', *Lancet*, 1886, 1, p.127.

56 Beard, *A Practical Treatise on Nervous Exhaustion*, pp.49-50.

57 Ibid., pp.124-5.

58 Ibid., p.155.

he estimated comprised one in ten of his patients, had been accused, 'very unjustly', of causing many to become addicted, but he could only say that, whilst there was something in 'the charge that opium-eating is caused by over prescribing', whatever was 'given as medicine, oftentimes becomes repulsive'.[59] Neurasthenia, then, was a physiological illness arising from a weakening of the 'nerve force' or 'nervous diathesia', a theory fundamentally similar to Thomas Trotter's notion of 'nervous temperament' formulated in 1807. But in this case it was placed on a scientific footing in the context of evolution and helped to prove the validity of then dominant social theories.

Many influential figures, for example William and Alice James, Charlotte Perkins Gilman, George Eliot, Max Weber, and Immanuel Kant were said to have suffered from the disease. Kant, an influential figure in the move towards philosophy within the proto-science of psychiatry, attributed many of these disturbances of the mind and emotions, and of human senses and their aberrations, to the march of civilisation. The growing complexities of progress were seen as a threat to well-being, to personal freedom and so to psychological health.[60] Friedrich Nietzsche understood the neurasthenic condition to be emblematic of the internalised guilt, and a glorification of the powerlessness, that he found at the centre of modern culture. Emile Durkheim recognised its manifestation as an explanatory metaphor for the violent changes of the age. Dr William Marrs, in publishing *Confessions of a Neurasthenic* (1887), *pace* De Quincey, made it decidedly fashionable for the great and the good to move in elite neurasthenic circles, displaying their martyrdom to their heightened sensibilities.[61]

Those who had the apparent misfortune to be manual workers rather than 'brain-workers' had traditionally, in medical and lay terms, failed to suffer from 'nervous debility'. In his *Anatomy of Melancholy* (1621) Richard Burton had asserted that the 'hired servant ... kept hard to her work and bodily labour' was never 'troubled in this kind', but 'noble virgins, nice gentlemen, such as are solitary and idle ... are misaffected and prone to this disease'. Thomas Sydenham had also observed that all were prone to suffer, bar those who 'lead a hard and hardy life', and in the early eighteenth century Mandeville was in agreement as to the susceptibility of the 'sedentary and luxury-laden classes'.[62] Roy Porter, discussing the decades around 1800, argues that anxieties about health were whipped up by physicians cashing in on new advances and opportunities, and creating what was derided by some of their contemporaries as the 'sick trade'. The Romantic idea that 'the world is too

---

59 Beard, *Stimulants and Narcotics*, pp.152-3.

60 Veith, *Hysteria*, pp.188, 192.

61 Lutz, *American Nervousness*, pp.4, 6, 23-4; Gosling, *Before Freud*, pp.x, 15.

62 Quoted in M.S. Micale, *Approaching Hysteria: Disease and its Interpretations* (1995), pp.154-5.

much with us' drove some to nervous distraction by 'pressures of wealth, ambition, emulation and self-deceit'.[63]

Nervousness had the historical reputation, and Beardian Neurasthenia a contemporary one, of being a highly respectable and now exciting and covetably elite disease to contract. Indeed Beard referred to neurasthenia as being 'distinguished' and as the 'unexplored Central Africa of medicine'. The 'miseries of the rich, the comfortable, and the intelligent', he argued, had so far been 'unstudied and unrelieved'.[64] Resting on its aetiology, rather than on a precise knowledge of any recognised pathology, neurasthenia as a single-disease concept was an all-encompassing condition heavily reliant on cultural biases and doctored to produce a viable scientific fact. Beard's theory of addiction enlisted the empiricism and scientific knowledge of men such as Anstie and imposed on it a rancorous blend of social science and theological ideology.

In his *Practical Treatise on Nervous Exhaustion*, however, Beard expressed the opinion that his work was a positive contribution to sociology in that it encompassed discussion of race, type, institutions and social customs. It did provide a respectable specialist vein of medical research and treatment and allowed for a broad and intermediate range of psychopathologies, and for the medicalisation of areas of mental life which would be fully monopolised in the twentieth century by the study of neuroses.[65] Defending his work, which had been worthy of criticism in the *Times* and the *Spectator*, against allegations that it was all a 'figment of the imagination', he profitably drew on the credibility of authorities such as Herbert Spencer.[66]

The Philosopher

> *No one can be perfectly free till all are free; no one can be perfectly moral till all are moral; no one can be perfectly happy till all are happy.*
>
> Herbert Spencer, *Social Statics*

As a systematic philosopher-scientist and cultural evolutionist, Herbert Spencer applied functional analysis to the individual and to society as a whole, and was amongst the first to suggest that human society could be studied scientifically. As such he was a leading figure in the nineteenth-century intellectual revolution.[67] Spencer's central tenet was that causation operates in human behaviour just as it does

---

63 R. Porter, 'Medicine', in McCalman, *Oxford Companion to the Romantic Age*, pp.173-4.

64 Beard, *Nervous Exhaustion*, pp.x, 8.

65 Micale, *Approaching Hysteria*, p.98; Scull, *The Most Solitary of Afflictions*, p.256, n.110.

66 Beard, *Stimulants and Narcotics*, p.114; *The Problems of Insanity* (1880), p.10.

67 J.H. Turner, *Herbert Spencer: A Renewed Appreciation* (1985); D.L. Sills, ed., *International Encyclopaedia of the Social Sciences* (1968-), pp.121-8.

in other spheres of nature. His belief in the inheritance of acquired characteristics as the major causal factor in organic evolution meant that, essentially, his biological theory directly informed his social theory, even after Darwin's explication of the mechanism of natural selection in 1859.[68]

In his *The Principles of Psychology* (1870) Spencer included an appendix entitled 'On the Actions of Anaesthetics and Narcotics'.[69] Here he elucidated accepted medical understanding of the actions of drugs and discussed the changes and anomalies within the nervous centres that he maintained determined the resultant psychical phenomena, and hence the propensity towards addiction. He acknowledged the common supposition that these drugs acted through special relations to particular nervous tissue, but wanted to expose what he considered to be the erroneous assumption arising from this that they therefore had affinities with very particular nervous centres. This assumption arose from the variety of effects which might be produced by a particular drug, when for example 'one drunken man becomes morose while another becomes affectionate', and was made, as Anstie had pointed out, only because it had served to make those effects intelligible. Spencer argued that the effect of a narcotic was comprehensible only as, by 'diffusion and re-diffusion', the drug was carried through the nervous system as a whole. This process explained the quandary as to why stimulation might precede narcosis and why different effects and consequences could then be observed in different individuals.

Spencer spelt out the process. As a narcotic was carried through the body each 'nerve-corpuscle' was thought to be quickly acted upon, and, as successive molecular transformations were wrought in it there resulted a 'general exaltation of state; as shown physically in the invigorated pulse and contractions of the muscles, and as shown psychically in the rush of vivid ideas and intensified feelings'. As the drug arrested the function of the nerve, it served, at the moment of its action, to excite the nerve, but it was then disabled and the symptoms of narcosis were produced. A small quantity of a drug would therefore have a stimulating effect little qualified by the narcotic effect, whereas a larger quantity would allow the narcosis to dominate. So, these drugs, 'swallowed or inhaled or injected, differ in their minor results [but] *do* agree in their major results as being excitants or sedatives according to circumstances, and as habitually producing exaltation of function before depression of function'.[70] It was these feelings of exaltation and depression, artificially induced but acting on the existing raw material, which, he explained, were the physiological bases of addiction.

The Principles of Psychology also included a chapter on 'Pleasures and Pains', *pace* De Quincey, in which Spencer addressed the aetiology of the condition of craving. His depiction of this 'pain', or 'discomfort', as a negative of 'pleasure' was rooted in his functional determinism. 'Pleasures and Pains' completed Spencer's

---

68 G. Jones, *Social Darwinism and English Thought: The Interaction between Biological and Social Theory* (1980), p.73.

69 Herbert Spencer, *The Principles of Psychology* (1870), 1, pp.272-88.

70 Ibid.

inductions of mental phenomena in this work and he referred to it as being 'perhaps the most obscure and involved which Psychology includes'. Addiction, involving a complex relationship between both pleasures and pain, was particularly opaque even though the science of psychology, aiming to be more than merely a science of consciousness, was rooted in empirical biology and the work of men such as Anstie. The subject matter of psychology was 'human experience considered as dependent upon the experiencing person' and the *raison d'être* of the psychologist was to observe this experience and to distinguish it from the observation of physical science. It was the 'translation of mental processes into words' which might provide an alternative or complimentary explanation for conditions such as addiction.[71]

In discussing the sensations of pleasure and pain, Spencer contented himself with setting down 'what appear to be the essentials'. The schema he constructed divided types of feelings into categories of agreeable and disagreeable, which, he acknowledged, traversed 'all other lines of demarkation'.[72] Nevertheless, Spencer did not baulk at putting forward a scientific explanation for the esoteric nature of these phenomena and at the same time provided a coherent analysis of a theory of addiction.

In his systematic approach pleasures and pains are described as concomitants of certain states, both local and general. These were particular and did not include all living states, some of which yielded to no consciousness of feeling at all and others, such as an ordinary sensation of touch, which were neither pleasurable nor painful. Spencer's logical question then, was 'what are the states which yield Pains and what are the states which yield Pleasures?' Certain pains, he argued, arose from states of inaction, and were called pains inasmuch as they were seen as antithetical to pleasures. These were the feelings best known as cravings.

Cravings due to the inaction of what Spencer termed higher 'epi-peripheral' feelings were classed as being relatively weak ones. They included, for example, sensations of touch, and as these were taken as being incessant, an agonising lack of them could never be experienced. Sound also came into this category and, also being 'habitual' and heard everywhere, he asserted that few ever felt the desire for it that followed continued silence. The argument was that a craving for light, colour or sound could only be felt after a period of confinement or sensory deprivation. The deprivation of the olfactory senses, however, was not seen in itself as a source of craving, though the desire for some natural tastes such as sweetness, and the still more 'acquired tastes' of alcohol and tobacco, did become persistent following the absence of odours. But these desires did not compare to the far stronger 'ento-peripheral' cravings with which they could often be confused.

These were powerful desires including, for example, muscular inaction, hunger and thirst which could become distinct discomforts and lead to an increasing intensity of painful feelings. Forms of emotional distress, 'the yearnings of the affections ... caused by the breaking of [the] closer human relations', *pace* Jones, were explained

71 Hardcastle, *What We Don't Know About Brains*, pp.92, 97-8.

72 Spencer, *Principles of Psychology*, pp.272-8.

as being, initially, 'certain inactions of the central organs of the nervous system', and in their full intensity as being a consciousness derived from the 'representation of a future in which such cravings will never be satisfied'. These were also seen as ento-peripheral pains, and of a similar nature to these terrible cravings were those that Spencer termed the 'abnormal appetites for habitual stimulants'.[73]

But these needs were pains born of inaction and they had opposite ones caused by excessive behaviour. The idea that the pleasures of excess might also be felt as pains showed a 'perceived approach to this effect of excess', and Spencer maintained that if a pain so caused was ever actually reached it would be a very rare experience indeed. So, in Spencer's analysis, there existed two extremes, 'the negative pains of inactions, called cravings, and ... the positive pains of excessive actions'. The implication was that pleasure only accompanied any action which fell between these extremes, that pleasure was the concomitant of 'medium activities'. According to this scientific schema, pleasure could only truly be experienced through moderate behaviour, even if it was admitted that that particular concept was mutable and might prove difficult to define. Spencer still had to ask himself the rhetorical questions: 'what constitutes a medium activity?' and 'what determines that lower limit of pleasurable action below which there is craving, and that higher limit of pleasurable action above which there is pain?'[74]

He searched for answers in an arena that had not yet been explored by psychologists, and turned to examine the conditions of the past under which, he argued, human feelings had been evolved. His argument for extreme states, positive and negative, led to the proposition that the medium state, where pleasure was experienced, was consistent with, or demanded by, a 'due balance of the functions constituting health'. That state was a natural, beneficial, almost political, 'guidance' conducive to the maintenance of life and to the success of longer-lived descendants. Thus, any excessive or defective behaviour was a detrimental disturbance of the '*consensus*' and that the 'general doctrine of Evolution [was] that pleasures are the incentives to life-supporting acts and pains the deterrents from life-destroying acts'.[75]

The presence of Spencer's 'moralistic view of the good society' is palpable in his language here, if not overtly stated.[76] His theory of 'equilibration' described cyclical processes in the social, organic and psychological realms that followed the course of evolution: of fluctuation in precarious equilibrium leading to eventual dissolution. The 'abnormal appetites' Spencer described were elements in this universal process of decay, and he maintained that if such 'ill-fitted' individuals were 'allowed to disappear' they would no longer be 'enabled to multiply at the expense of the capable and industrious'. In addressing the problem of why some individuals might develop such detrimental appetites, Spencer argued that these 'derangements' were due to an 'enforced persistence in habits of life at variance with the needs of the constitution'.

73 Ibid.

74 Ibid.

75 Ibid.

76 Turner, *Herbert Spencer*, p.34.

People, for example, daily forced by circumstance into 'undue and painful action' will be liable eagerly to indulge themselves to excess in any pleasures they can when they can get them. Responsibility for addiction lay with society as well as with the individual.

It was axiomatic, according to Spencer, that pleasures and pains could be acquired, 'as it were, superposed on certain feelings which did not originally yield them'. That is, various substances found at first to be distasteful could become pleasurable with persistent indulgence and the effects of habit. No argument was offered that pain could be 'superposed' on feelings originally agreeable, but he stated that 'we have proof that the state of consciousness called disgust may be made inseparable from a feeling that was once pleasurable'. He considered it probable that 'nearly everyone can furnish from his own experience some instance of acquired aversion'.[77]

Spencer maintained, in accordance with general contemporary liberal beliefs, that 'everyone is at liberty to do what he desires to do', but he considered this notion incomplete and illusory. He argued that the real proposition was whether everyone was at liberty to desire or not to desire. If, as he maintained, an individual were constituted from an aggregate of his feelings and ideas, and that his conscious self was inseparable from these psychical states, then to say that the performance of an action was the result of his free will was to say that he determined the mix of psychical states which aroused the action. Since these states constituted the individual, to say that they determined themselves was, he conjectured, absurd.[78] What he called 'the desire to perform [an] act' was a composite psychical state derived from ideal sensory impressions representing distant consequences. Feelings, then, such as cravings, that were 'immediately derived from the senses or mediately suggested by such', produced nascent ideal motor changes which would tend to inspire or to prevent the desire being fulfilled. If an immense number of psychical states were partially aroused, some would unite with the original impression in exciting the action, while the rest would combine to prevent action. When an accumulated stimulus became sufficiently powerful the nascent motor changes would become actual. The Will came into existence through the increasing complexity and imperfect coherence of these automatic actions. This was implied by the converse in that when actions once incoherent and voluntary were frequently repeated, they became coherent and involuntary and took the form of habit or addiction. Any set of psychical changes would then cease to be conscious, rational, and emotional and, by constant repetition, they would pass beyond the sphere of volition. This, according to Spencer, was not only the case with everyday actions, but was also particularly so 'with special habits'.

77 Spencer, *Principles of Psychology*, pp.272-8.

78 Ibid., pp.498-502.

Concluding remarks

The formation of predominant paradigms of formal knowledge was necessary for a professional acceptance of all medical concepts within science, and Anstie, Beard and Spencer all had their influential parts to play in this process. Anstie's taxonomy of drugs and drug reactions, Beard's construction of the disease-entity of neurasthenia, and Spencer's elucidation of the principles of psychology all embraced the concept of addiction. Anstie understood it as a mechanical, sometimes self-imposed deviation from an ideal physiological state of health, but not a 'special disease of the nervous system'. To Beard it was certainly just this, and eminently and profitably treatable, its aetiology differing according to the individual crasis of the sufferer, most importantly resting on hereditary type. Spencer, too, argued that addiction was an inherently physiological condition, but did not designate it as a disease. It took the form, he believed, of an eventual and complete suspension of the Will, the result of repetitive action at variance with the constitution, the will itself emanating from and dependent upon physiological balance. These conceptual schemes drew and elaborated upon common stocks of knowledge, they differed in language and formulation, but they all brought addiction firmly within the confined parameters of medical science and social vilification.

The idea that science might provide a determining role in human behaviour allowed the possibility of a world that could operate in a 'harmonious and morally elevated' way, a world which could perhaps, as Spencer suggested, aspire to a creative evolution and become a perfect society. Such positivism, however, denied dearly held ideas of rationality, individuality and autonomy, and it removed self-control and freedom, qualities highly regarded and cherished as virtues in Victorian ideology. Evident disgust was aroused by those, described in J. S. Mill's *On Liberty* (1859), 'whose desires and impulses [were] not [their] own', but also by those who were driven by habits and temptations and who therefore had 'no character, no more than a steam engine has a character'.[79] The amoral type, lacking in autonomy and self-control, was effectively a machine, dehumanised and potentially demonised. The fear of the abject nature of such a humiliating condition, a virtual death of the will, provoked feelings of disgust and anxiety and motivated the desire to understand and to 'cure'.

---

79 A. Anderson, *Tainted Souls and Painted Faces: The rhetoric of fallenness in Victorian culture* (1993), p.142.

Conclusion

The fairy tales of science, and the long result of time
Alfred Lord Tennyson, *Lockesly Hall*, 1.12

The use and abuse of opium in nineteenth-century Britain crossed gender, class, race and culture, and while personal accounts reveal that opium experiences remained essentially similar, attitudes to it continued to change. De Quincey's *Confessions*, with all its accumulated meanings and dark allusions, became an enduring part of the common idiom and was fully entrenched by the beginning of the twentieth century and beyond.[1] His account of the pleasures of opium, though couched in Romantic language, remains definitive:

> The ocean, in everlasting but gentle agitation, and brooded over by dove-like calm, might not unfitly typify the mind and the mood which then swayed it. For it seemed to me as if then first I stood at a distance, and aloof from the uproar of life; as if the tumult, the fever, and the strife, were suspended; a respite granted from the secret burthens of the heart; a sabbath of repose; a resting from human labours. Here were the hopes which blossom in the paths of life, reconciled with the peace which is in the grave; motions of the intellect as unwearied as the heavens, yet for all anxieties a halcyon calm: a tranquillity that seemed no product of inertia ... Oh! just, subtle, and mighty opium! ... bringest an assuaging balm ... a brief oblivion.[2]

A suicide letter, written at the beginning of the twentieth century, described the experience thus:

> When an opium-eater starts out on his career, each time he takes his daily dose in about half-an-hour the action of the heart increases, and that organ does double duty by sending the blood dancing through the veins ... The opium-eater feels a better man under its influence, and this without the brain becoming cloudy, as with liquor. The sensation is glorious ... it is for all the world as though some invisible hand was wrapping a warm blanket around that organ. No one can imagine the pleasure and strength – mentally and physically – that the drug gives.[3]

---

1 De Quincey's place in popular culture is illustrated by the actor, Gary Oldman, who played Sid Vicious in the film 'Sid and Nancy' in the 1990s. Oldman stated that he had taken De Quincey as a 'father figure' and role model for his portrayal of addiction. His characterisation had involved immersing himself in the *Confessions*. See E. Baxter, *De Quincey's Art of Autobiography* (1990), p.187, n.27.

2 De Quincey, *Confessions*, p.49.

3 *Pharmaceutical Journal*, August 25 1900, p.251.

The *Pharmaceutical Journal* printed the account, describing it as a suicide's 'Confessions', though it lacked 'the artistic quality attaching to those of De Quincey'. The author was a fifty-two-year-old shipping clerk who, having taken fifty to sixty grains of opium a day for fifteen years, was discovered comatose and alone in a boarding-house, dying two days later from his overdose. He had attempted suicide with 'half an ounce of laudanum, then one ounce, then one-eighth of an ounce of opium, then a quarter of an ounce, and, at last, three-eighths of an ounce of opium – but all without effect'. He finally achieved his aim with half an ounce of the solid drug, over three times his daily dose. Whilst his description of the blissful sensations of opium was similar to De Quincey's, he and his circumstances were not and the reaction of denigration and contempt was palpable. Modern accounts of opiate effects, produced in different settings again, concur: the sensation flows 'down over your body, warming, insulating, tingling, denying all pain, fear and sadness'. It is 'the mother of all things. It's a comforter, its puts its arms around you and embraces you [it] dims the lights and makes you nice and warm'.[4] But the twenty-first-century observer has his or her own assumptions about 'illicit', or illegal, opiate use, and they are based on a history of fear, ignorance and a need for control.

The nineteenth-century formation of a predominant paradigm of formal knowledge was necessary for a professional acceptance of the concept of addiction as a disease entity, but still there existed a clear and unbridgeable distinction between science and the mind. There remained an unease with the visionary effects of drugs and any suggestion of creative, mystical experience as described by De Quincey *et al.*, experiences that were still constantly alluded to throughout the late nineteenth century. It might be suggested that such subjective ideas and experiences required gainsaying because of the inability of science to measure them.

Connections between addiction, medicine, insanity, and the concept of 'vice' were already becoming familiar in the early nineteenth century. Controversy, anxiety and contempt had emanated from the tensions inherent in mind–body duality, and they remained and persisted as the physiological and psychological 'symptoms' of addiction were gradually enshrined in medical nosologies and practice. Since the mid-nineteenth century the addict has been portrayed as weak-willed, morally corrupt, degenerate, sociopathic, psychopathic, socially impoverished, a developmental failure, developmentally regressed, organically impaired, a subject of conditioning, a victim of political repression, and psychologically dependent.[5] It has been argued that science 'cannot increase our understanding of ourselves and our world ... if it is held captive by our fears', and empirical medicine was demonstrably unable to describe or explain the experience of addiction without descending into moral opprobrium, particularly where personal, political, ethical or economic interests were involved.[6]

---

4 T. Stewart, *The Heroin Users* (1987), p.36; N. McCormick, 'Junk Bonds', *The Observer Magazine*, 20 May 2001, pp.18-23.

5 Schaffer and Burglass, *Classic Contributions to the Addictions*, p.486.

6 Peele, *The Meaning of Addiction*, p.xii.

The works of De Quincey, Coleridge, Lamb and their peers had introduced a romantic sensibility enhanced by opium which was seized upon by the medical profession, involved as it was in a process of reform and specialisation. Initially physicians were most concerned with taxonomic works cataloguing the various drugs within the pharmacopoeia, but in discussing the properties and effects of opium they could not divorce empirical observation from moral comment. In 1836 the *Lancet* carried the text of a lecture on 'Materia Medica and Therapeutics' which reminded the audience that almost every physician, 'who has practised his profession for some time, has seen patients take, from being long habituated to its use, enormous quantities of laudanum, or solid opium', whilst a subsequent lecture stressed the abuse of the drug in a luxurious fashion, in suicides, and in accidental and deliberate poisonings.[7] Attitudes to chronic opium use changed from the perception of it as a creative sensibility and an intellectually stimulating experience to a reductive, self-destructive sickness.

Much of the medical involvement emanated from the struggle for status and professional recognition and involved a need to monopolise knowledge, means, and technique. Moral injunction was a tool in this process. The *Lancet*'s publication of research by the Analytical Sanitary Commission in 1854, which concentrated on opium and its adulterations, had, as an epigraph to each article, the telling phrase 'To attack vice in the abstract without attacking persons, may be safe fighting indeed, but it is fighting with shadows'.[8] The medical profession was already involved in a 'war' on opium which was seen to be a dangerous poison, an agent of vice, and often fatally destructive in the wrong, non-medical hands.

By the 1880s the 'evil' of opium was regarded as being safe only 'in the hands of medical men who appreciate its dangers' and 'abuse almost certainly followed' when it was used by an unsupervised public.[9] Seymour Sharkey, discussing opium abuse, declared himself 'convinced that the prevention of the evil rests rather with the public in general than with medical men'. Without medical control, addicts would, he believed, continue to 'poison themselves' and would be destroyed by an enfeeblement of the will which 'makes the man a moral paralytic, of all spectacles the most pitiable this side of the grave.[10] The medical profession, attempting to monopolise control of opium use, emphasised its poisonous nature and the lack of public restraint in the face of the drug. Articles on 'The great abuse of narcotics in all classes of society' appeared, discussing fashion and death in the same breath. Another on 'Remarks on Poisons as Used by the Medical Profession and Abused by the Public' castigated the excessive and diseased 'vice' of 'hundreds and thousands' of addicts, but asked the medical profession, 'are we not often ourselves to blame?'[11]

---

7 *Lancet*, 1836-37, 1, pp.354-5; 1837, 2, pp.785-94.

8 See for example: *Lancet*, 1854, 1, p.10.

9 S. Sharkey, 'Morphinomania', *The Nineteenth Century*, 1887, 22, pp.335-42.

10 Ibid., pp.339, 341, 342.

11 H. Barnes, 'On the Abuse of Narcotics', *British Medical Journal*, 25 November 1882, pp.1032-3; B. Marsack, 'Remarks on Poisons as Used by the Medical Profession and

A biomedical explanation of addiction provided answers to the condition and was a compelling argument for regulation of the drug. The implication was that because addiction seemed to have similar symptoms to some nineteenth-century mental illnesses, it too was a disease. But it was a murky condition with unknown causes and unknown cures; as such it was susceptible to symbolic embellishment and metaphorical analogies of the corruption and pollution of society, as well as the individual.[12] The disease metaphor had profound implications for the ways in which addiction was, and is now, conceptualised. The aetiology of, and treatments for, addiction were given over to biomedical approaches which still, today, continue to search for an answer to the disease of addiction, a disease which has consistently demonstrated a remarkable capacity to resist treatments.[13]

Medicine came to recognise distinct pathological responses to chronic opium use and constructed a disease entity around them with aetiology, symptoms and treatments. When the social and cognitive life of the addict was not taken into account, or was interpreted in the light of prejudice, then his or her addiction could be seen as qualitatively different from any other form of human desire and could be designated a disease. A purely biological concept of addiction, whilst it apparently provided a discrete and factual basis of understanding, was, on its own, virtually useless. But Herbert Spencer's theory of essential desires as being fundamental to the human condition included addiction, or 'craving', in his schema along with any other need. These desires were also the subject matter of psychology, 'the human experience considered as dependent upon the experiencing person', and as such he believed these experiences required an understanding other than that of physical science alone. Where 'Body and Gut' physicians, such as George Beard, were concerned, addiction was a physical symptom of a material world and it required physical treatments.

Faith in new medical science reflected the Victorian idea of progress, and came to be perceived as embodying the ability to cleanse: it could provide a unifying principle and give meaning to the idea of human progress in an increasingly secular environment. This faith, in what amounted to a cult of 'scientism', invested with credence by evolutionary theory, gave a foundation to an approach to the human condition which was observable and 'factual', and which aroused both lay and medical response.[14] The pervasiveness of such an ideology came to acquire a quite intoxicating fervour, and gave an explanation and legitimacy to certain social anxieties and their apparent remedies. Thus the 'luxurious' use of drugs, as with other forms of behaviour deemed dangerous and disorderly, could be seen as abhorrent to

---

Abused by the Public', *British Medical Journal*, 15 July 1882, pp.86-7.

12 S. Sontag, *Illness as Metaphor* (1979), passim.

13 G.A. Marlatt and K Fromme, 'Metaphors for Addiction', in S. Peele, ed., *Visions of Addiction: Major Contemporary Perspectives on Addiction and Alcoholism* (1988), pp.1-24.

14 A.R. Morris, 'Oscar Wilde and the Eclipse of Darwinianism: Aestheticism, Degeneration, and Moral Reaction in Late Victorian Ideology', *Studies in the History and Philosophy of Science*, 1993, 24, pp.513-40. Disease rhetoric, Morris argues, emerged strengthened from the debate over Darwin's *The Origin of the Species* (1859).

the very laws of nature and could be used to sanction the dominant moral code.[15] The apparent universality of the acceptance and centrality of such a code denied unorthodox behaviour such as drug taking for pleasure, and arguably created a lasting 'moral panic', particularly with the weight of ratiocinative scientism behind it.[16]

15 M. Douglas, *Purity and Danger: An analysis of the concepts of pollution and taboo* (1966), pp.3-4. Douglas posits that 'pollution ideas' operate in society on instrumental and expressive levels, and that exaggerating differences and separating, cleansing and punishing transgressions serves to impose order onto a potentially chaotic experience.

16 For a discussion of moral crises and the application of this model to 'marginal' behaviour see J. Weeks, *Sex, Politics and Society: The regulation of sexuality since 1800* (1989), p.14.

Appendix One

Opium Strengths and Doses

Approximate estimates of opium doses and strengths according to Goodman and Gillman, *The Pharmacological Basis of Therapeutics* (1996).

Liquid drops & ounces:

1 drop = 1/20 ml
20 drops = 1 ml
1 fluid ounce = 29.5 ml
1 fluid ounce = 590 drops
20 fluid ounces = 1 English pint

By weight:

[Goodman and Gillman took the figure of 1 grain of opium equalling 25 drops of laudanum from De Quincey's *Confessions*. A grain is the smallest British weight, the average weight of a seed of corn, about one seven thousandth of a pound.]

Opium = 10% morphine
25 drops laudanum = 1 grain opium = 64 mg opium
1 grain opium = 64 mg opium = 6.4 mg morphine
1 liquid ounce laudanum = 590 drops laudanum
590 drops laudanum = 23 ¾ grains opium
23 ¾ grains opium = 1,520 mg opium
1,520 mg opium = 152 mg morphine

Therefore:
1 liquid ounce laudanum = 152 mg morphine
1 English pint laudanum = 3,040 mg morphine = 3.04 grams

Cost:

[According to Berridge in *Opium and the People* (1981) laudanum was sixpence an ounce in the early nineteenth century.]

1 ounce laudanum = sixpence
20 ounces laudanum = 1 pint = 10 shillings
7 pints a week = daily dose 3 grams morphine = average weekly cost £3 10s = average annual cost £182

Goodman and Gillman suggest that the tolerance of a confirmed drug addict can run as high as 5 grams of morphine a day. According to Southey, Coleridge regularly took at least 'two quarts of laudanum a week, the cost of which is £5, and sometimes he swallowed a pint a day', which means he was sometimes taking just over 3 grams of morphine, costing an astonishing 10 shillings a day.

Appendix Two

Opium and Alcohol

Alcoholism has been ably and thoroughly explored elsewhere, notably by such as Harrison, Porter, Bynum, McLeod and Pruitt, and I do not intend to trespass there except to briefly note the parallels drawn by users of opium and alcohol and by nineteenth-century physicians, and to point to comparative arguments used by pro- and anti-opium campaigners.[1] Harrison argues that alcohol was an important ubiquitous pain-killer and that the 'Victorians often failed to distinguish between alcoholism, drinking and drunkenness'.[2] As with opium there was confusion and controversy over whether a certain behaviour was a disease, a habitual vice, or a pleasurable pursuit.

Opium and alcohol have historically been used in parallel in medical practice as well as in sensual pursuits. Late eighteenth- and early nineteenth-century medical texts on alcohol prefigured those on opiates in arguing that addiction be recognised as a disease. One of the most prominent of these works was Benjamin Rush's *An Inquiry into the Effects of Ardent Spirits Upon the Human Body and Mind* (1785).[3] Rush proposed a 'Moral and Physical Thermometer', a form of drinker's progress which depicted the drinking of water as producing 'Serenity of Mind, Reputation, Long Life, & Happiness', and, at the other end of the imbiber's spectrum, the taking of 'Drams of Gin, Brandy, and Rum' morning, noon and night as invariably inducing vices such as 'Stealing & Swindling, Perjury, Burglary, and Murder'. The confirmed drinker would inevitably descend into 'Melancholy, Madness and Despair', ending up in Bridewell or on the gallows. Rush's work, and others such as Thomas Trotter's *Essay, Medical, Philosophical, and Chemical, on Drunkenness* (1804), were concerned with the concept of habit as a physiological 'disease of the mind' and as

---

1 B. Harrison, *Drink and the Victorians: The Temperance Question in England 1815-1872* (1971); W.F. Bynum, 'Chronic alcoholism in the first half of the nineteenth century', *Bulletin of the History of Medicine*, 1968, xlii, pp.160-85; R. Porter, 'The drinking man's disease: the pre-history of alcoholism in Georgian Britain', *British Journal of Addiction*, 1985, 80, pp.385-96; R. McLeod, 'The edge of hope: social policy and chronic alcoholism, 1870-1900', *Journal of the History of Medicine*, July 1967, pp.215-45; A. Pruitt, 'Approaches to alcoholism in mid-Victorian Britain', *Clio Medica*, 1974, 9, pp.93-101.

2 Harrison, *Drink and the Victorians*, pp.23, 42.

3 Rush, an American, had studied medicine at Edinburgh and his ideas had enormous influence in both Britain and in America, where he took a leading role in the Temperance movement. He was politically eminent, elected to the Continental Congress, a signatory of the Declaration of Independence and, later, Treasurer of the US Mint. Perhaps most importantly he is seen as the founder of psychiatry in America.

a question of will. Although Rush argued that the drunkard might be no more able to control his drinking than he could control a convulsive movement of his limbs, a belief echoed by Coleridge who was probably familiar with Rush's work, he could not divorce the behaviour from moral arguments.

Addiction might encompass any habit-forming substance and De Quincey, in his *Confessions*, addressed what he saw as a misleading lack of distinction between the effects of alcohol and opium.[4] Anxious to dismiss any vulgar suggestion of similarity, he maintained that alcohol disordered the mind with base sensuality whilst opium brought clarity, grace and truth. But the parallels were always there, both drugs intoxicated and were known to lead to habitual use in some.

Charles Lamb's *Confessions of a Drunkard* had prefigured De Quincey's admissions of habit by eight years, being first published in the Utilitarian magazine, the *Philanthropist*, in 1813.[5] The essay was reprinted in Basil Montague's book, *Some Enquiries into the Effects of Fermented Liquors* in 1814, and next reappeared in the *London Magazine* in 1822, hot on the heels of De Quincey's *Confessions*. Lamb's piece gave an account of the pleasures of drink which entrapped his young, weak and nervous self, but it dwelt on the pains of his long addiction. He analogously described a print, after Correggio, in which:

> three female figures are ministering to a man who sits fast bound at the root of a tree. Sensuality is soothing him, Evil Habit is nailing him to a branch, and Repugnance is … applying a snake to his side. In his face is feeble delight, the recollection of past rather than perception of present pleasures … a submission to bondage.[6]

To attempt to break his addiction would have been to walk 'through fire', to have been 'flayed alive', and to 'undergo a change violent as that which we conceive of the mutation of form in some insects'.[7] It has been suggested that alcohol to Lamb was as opium to Coleridge, 'a deadening of the pain of living … a solvent of speech'.[8] Lamb himself, having resolved to abstain, had asked 'is life, with such limitations, worth trying?'[9] By 1831 the question of insanity had arisen. Thomas Carlyle had written that he sincerely believed Lamb to be 'in some considerable degree *insane* … a confirmed and shameless drunkard [who] *asks* vehemently for gin-and-water in strangers' houses'.[10] The word opium could, without argument, replace alcohol in any of these experiences and responses. It is addiction that they describe.

---

4 See chapter 2, p.27.

5 The editors of the *Philanthropist* were the Benthamite James Mill and the Quaker James Allen. The sub-title of the magazine was 'Repository for Hints and Suggestions calculated to promote the Comfort and Happiness of Man'.

6 Lamb, C., *Confessions of a Drunkard* (1st. published 1813), in Phillips, A., ed., *Charles Lamb: Selected Prose* (1985), pp.155-61.

7 Ibid.

8 R.L. Hine, *Charles Lamb and his Hertfordshire* (1849), p.310.

9 Levine, *The Romantic Art of Confession*, pp.83-4.

10 Ibid.

Publishing his *Confessions* was a risky and potentially self-damaging act for Lamb, at that time a lowly clerk. His drinking habits were well known and, in the 1822 publication, he thought it necessary to add a coda which, though it did not deny 'that a portion of his own experiences may have passed into the picture', laid the most part of the work at the door of the imagination. Nonetheless he defensively thought it 'useless to expostulate' with 'cold, washy, spiteful, bloodless … slime', who had 'watery heads with hearts of jelly'. He would humiliate his critics, he protested, with satire, and expose their vapid self-righteousness with 'his long promised, but unaccountably hitherto delayed, *Confessions of a Water-drinker*'.[11]

The medical profession sheltered every argument and opinion in the debates over the merits or otherwise of opium and alcohol. William Carpenter, the recipient of one hundred guineas for his prize-winning essay *On the Use and Abuse of Alcoholic Liquors in Health and Disease*, published in the *Lancet* in 1849, recommended the apparently invulnerable position of 'Total Abstinence'. Quoting Archdeacon Jeffreys of Bombay he self-righteously insisted that, out of all the 'gifts of Providence [and] all the enjoyments of life ... there is not one of them which the wickedness of man does not more or less abuse'. Other physicians held a less dogmatic point of view and were prepared to concede that the question might be one of degree and choice of drug. James Maxwell declared that 'once the [opium] *habit* is contracted, so tight is the hold it takes upon a man', that he would find it almost impossible to break, whereas the '*ordinary* consumer of alcoholic liquors requires no such help in giving them up'. 'Whoever heard', he asked, 'of the *ordinary* beer-drinker coming to a doctor for help in order to give up his beer? The two practices are not to be compared in respect of the intensity of the grasp exercised by the two drugs respectively upon the *moderate* consumer'.[12]

Edward Harper Parker, however, a consulate official in China in the 1860s and 70s much concerned with the opium trade, suggested that 'much less harm is done by opium-smoking than is done by strong drink in Great Britain … never once have I seen an opium-smoker take the angry and self-justificatory attitude which some of our advocates of free drink will do.' In China the 'casual observer' of opium use sees

> very little of the horrors which undoubtedly do occasionally take place [yet] which of us is not a frequent witness in the cities of Great Britain to the ruin and misery caused by excessive indulgence in strong drink? From what I have personally observed … of drink on the one hand and opium on the other … the impression left upon me is very distinct that opium does much less harm … than drink … so far as inciting to acts of violence, neglect of family, &c., are concerned.[13]

11 Phillips, *Charles Lamb*, pp.411-12.

12 *British Medical Journal*, 2 July 1881, p.30.

13 E.H. Parker, 'Personal Reminiscences touching Opium-Smoking', *Blackwood's Edinburgh Magazine*, April 1896, pp.576, 579.

Letter writers to the *Times* in the 1880s agreed: opium users were only a 'nuisance ... from lingering so long in a state of harmless dullness'. They existed in a passive state, 'satisfied with [their] own dreamy condition ... useless, but not mischievous. It is quite otherwise with alcoholic liquors'.[14] Conceding that 'opium taken internally was a powerful and dangerous narcotic stimulant' he argued that it was 'no worse in the effects produced by excessive use than alcohol'. On the contrary alcohol, 'in the production of crime and brutal violence of every kind', filled the prisons and fed the gallows:

> Nothing has ever been said of opium that can equal the evil which has been written and spoken of strong drinks. Judges from the Bench, and preachers from the pulpit, vie with each other in denouncing this as a national vice ... [and] lament their powerlessness to stop its terrible ravages. The clergy declare it to be the most formidable stumbling-block in the way of Christianity. We are told that nine-tenths of the 40,000 prisoners in our jails are there for crimes committed under the influence of drink; and in a paper by Dr. Norman Kerr, read lately at the Social Science Congress, the annual mortality from drink is estimated at 128,000, while the number of habitual drunkards reaping this harvest of death and misery to all belonging to them, is put at 600,000.[15]

The correspondents rebuffed the objection that opium was a designated poison by Act of Parliament and declared that alcohol was obviously a poison too, deemed to be so by no less than medical expertise and popular consensus. Sir William Gull, speaking to the Lord's Committee on alcohol had remarked that 'a very large number of people in society are dying day by day, poisoned by alcoholic drinks' and he 'hardly knew any more powerful source of disease'. It was a question, he believed, of urging philanthropists to tackle this problem 'of colossal proportions ... at their own door', before turning their attention and efforts to the opium trade.[16] These arguments were undoubtedly factional, the weight of political and commercial interests were clearly making themselves felt, but the opinions expressed reveal much about attitudes to addictions. It was a moveable feast: one could be compassionate and liberal, or disgusted and punitive according to the drug, the addict and the perceptions and interests of the observer.

The Reverend E.E. Jenkins, speaking at an anti-opium meeting in Mansion House in 1881, agreed in principle with the medical profession that 'opium is poison'. Those who endeavoured to 'liken the consumption of it to the use of alcoholic beverages in this country, know not what they say ... outside the medical necessity it is a ruthless and an indiscriminating destroyer of body and of mind'.[17] But he begged to make a professional, partisan and moral distinction. In his opinion the 'insidious danger' of alcohol was that it was 'rather a luxury than a poison' and therefore carried a moral

---

14 Letters to the *Times*, 26 December 1881 and 20 January 1882 reprinted in Sultzberger, *All About Opium*, pp.23, 82.

15 Ibid.

16 Ibid., pp.62-6.

17 Sultzberger, *All About Opium*, p.10.

opprobrium far greater than its potential for physiological harm. Opium could still perhaps be kept within the control of the profession and so was regarded, 'from first to last', as a drug and a poison: 'its proper place is in medicine, and there only'.[18] Opinion and interest in the nineteenth century were divided on the use and abuse of alcohol and of opium much as they are today. Harrison, for example, argues that the 'free-licensing argument has much in common with the present-day case for deregulating the drug trade'.[19] What differs is that *addiction* has, through those arguments, come to be understood as a discrete condition regardless of whichever substance or behaviour it is that results in its manifestation.

18 *Lancet*, 1886, 1, p.891.

19 Harrison, *Drink and the Victorians*, p.64. That is that high prices, demand, adulteration and smuggling can be eliminated by, in the case of drugs, legalisation and 'free competition'. The problems 'flourish only when government regulation lends [drug-taking] an artificial attraction.'

Bibliography

Primary Literature

Books

Allbutt, T.C., and Dixon, W.E., *A System of Medicine* (London, 1906).

Anon., *Poppies: a talk with English boys and girls about opium* (London, 1860).

Anstie, F.E., *Stimulants and Narcotics: Their Mutual Relations* (London, 1864).

Baillie, J., *The Dramatic and Poetical Works* (London, 1851).

Beard, G.M., *Stimulants and Narcotics: Medically, Philosophically, and Morally Considered* (NY, 1871).

———, *A Practical Treatise on Nervous Exhaustion (Neurasthenia), its Symptoms, Nature, Sequences, Treatment* (NY, 1880).

Blackmore, R., *A Treatise of the Spleen and Vapours* (London, 1726).

Bram Stoker, *Dracula* (London, 1897).

Brontë, A., *The Tenant of Wildfell Hall*, Panther edition 1969 (1st published London, 1848).

Brooks, M.G., *Judith, Esther, and Other Poems* (London, 1820).

Christison, R., *Of the Action of Opium and the Symptoms it Excites in Man* (Edinburgh, 1827).

———, *On Poisons* (Edinburgh, 1829).

———, *A Treatise on Poisons in Relation to Medical Jurisprudence, Physiology, and the Practice of Physic* (Edinburgh, 1829).

Crumpe, S., *An Inquiry into the Nature and Properties of Opium* (London, 1793).

Collins, W., *The Moonstone, A Romance* (Penguin edition 1994. 1st published London, 1868).

———, *The Woman in White* (Penguin edition 1974. 1st published London, 1860).

Conan-Doyle, A., *The Sign of Four*, in *The Original Illustrated 'Strand' Sherlock Holmes* (London, 1887).

De Quincey, T., *Confessions of an English Opium Eater* (London, 1821. OUP, 1985).

Dickens, Charles, *Bleak House* (London, 1853).

———, *Hard Times* (Penguin 1982. 1st published London, 1854).

———, *The Mystery of Edwin Drood* (London, Penguin edition 1974. 1st published London, 1870).

Doré, G., and Jerrold, W.B., *London, A Pilgrimage* (London, 1872).

Dowden, E., ed., *The correspondence of Robert Southey with Caroline Bowles. To which are added: correspondence with Shelley, and Southey's dreams* (London, 1881).

Eliot, George, *Silas Marner, The Weaver of Raveloe* (London, 1861).

———,*Middlemarch* (Penguin edition 1994. 1st published London, 1871-72).

———,*Felix Holt, The Radical* (Penguin edition 1987. 1st published London, 1866).

———,*Daniel Deronda* (Penguin edition 1967. 1st published London, 1876).

Greenwood, J., *In Strange Company* (London, 1883).

Gosse, E., *In Russet and Silver* (London, 1894).

Hogg, J., *De Quincey and His Friends: personal recollections, souvenirs, and anecdotes of Thomas De Quincey, his friends and associates* (London, 1895).

Jennings, O., *On the Cure of the Morphia Habit* (London, 1890).

———, *On the Cure of the Morphia Habit Without Suffering* (London, 1901).

———, *The Morphia habit and its Voluntary Renunciation (A personal relation of a suppression after twenty-five years' addiction). With notes and additional cases* (London, 1909).

Jones, J., *The Mysteries of Opium Reveal'd* (London, 1700).

Kerr, N., *Inebriety, its Etiology, Pathology, Treatment, and Jurisprudence* (London, 1888).

Kingsley, Charles, *Alton Locke* (London, 1851).

Nisbet, J.F., *The insanity of genius and the general inequality of human faculty psychologically considered* (London, 1881).

Lloyd, Charles, *Edmund Oliver* (London, 1798).

Richardson, B.W., *Diseases of Modern Life* (London, 1876).

Rush, B., *An Enquiry into the Effects of Spiritous Liquors on the Human Body* (Edinburgh, 1791).

Sainsbury, H., *Drugs and the Drug Habit* (London, 1909).

Spencer, H., *Principles of Psychology* (London, 1870).

Sultzberger, H., ed., *All About Opium* (London, 1884).

Taylor, A.S., *On Poisons in Relation to Medical Jurisprudence and Medicine* (London, 1848).

Trotter, T., *An Essay, Medical, Philosophical, and Chemical, on Drunkenness, and its Effects on the Human Body* (London, 1804).

Wilde, O., *The Picture of Dorian Gray* (Wordsworth edition 1992. 1st published London, 1891).

Articles (Some items not listed here will have been too numerous to include and instead are fully listed in the text, as in the case of the Lancet and British Medical Journal.)

Allbutt, T.C., 'On the abuse of hypodermic injections of morphia', *Practitioner* (1870) 5, pp.327-31.

Anon., 'In an opium den', *Ragged School Union*, September (1863) 20, pp.198-200.

———, 'East London Opium Smokers', *London Society* (1868) 14, pp.68-72.

———, 'What the Chinese think about opium', *The Friend of China*, October (1875) pp.195-7.

Christison, R., 'Article X, Cases and Observations in Medical jurisprudence – Case X On the Effects of Opium-Eating on Health and Longevity', *Edinburgh Medical and Surgical Journal* (1832) 17.

Hogarth, J.E., 'Literary Degenerates', *The Fortnightly Review* (1895) 57, pp.586-92.

Mattison, J.B., 'Opium addiction among medical men', *Medical Record* (1883) 23, pp.621-3.

Sharkey, S., 'Morphinomania', *Nineteenth Century*, September (1887) 22, pp.335-42.

Periodicals

Times
Gentleman's Magazine
Strand magazine
Friend of China
London Society
Chemist and Druggist
Practitioner
Eclectic Magazine
Blackwood's Magazine
Nineteenth Century
Lancet
British Medical Journal
Bell's Pharmaceutical Journal
Edinburgh Medical and Surgical Journal
Medico-Chirurgical Review and Journal
Pall Mall Gazette

Secondary Literature

Books

Abel, E.L., *A Dictionary of Drug Abuse Terms and Terminology* (London, 1984).

Ageyev, M., *Novel With Cocaine* (London, 1999).

Anderson, A., *Tainted Souls and Painted Faces: The Rhetoric of Fallenness in Victorian Culture* (Cornell University, 1993).

Anderson, O., *Suicide in Victorian and Edwardian England* (OUP, 1987).

Armstrong, T., Campbell, M., & Vice, S., eds, *Beyond the Pleasure Dome: Writing and addiction from the Romantics* (London, 1994).

Bakalar, J.B., and Grinspoon, L., *Marihuana: The Forbidden Medicine* (Yale University Press, 1993).

Baker, R., Porter, D., and Porter, R., eds, *The Codification of Medical Morality: Historical and Philosophical Studies of the Formalization of Western Medical Morality in the Eighteenth and Nineteenth Centuries*, vol.1, 'Medical Ethics and Etiquette in the Eighteenth Century' (London, 1993).

Batts, J.S., *British Manuscript Diaries of the Nineteenth Century: An annotated listing* (London, 1976).

Baxter, E., *De Quincey's Art of Autobiography* (Edinburgh, 1990).

Berridge, V., and Edwards, G., *Opium and the People: Opiate Use in Nineteenth-Century England* (London, 1981).

Blumberg, J., *Byron and the Shelleys: The Story of a Friendship* (London, 1992).

Blunden, E., *Charles Lamb, His Life. Recorded by his Contemporaries* (London, 1934).

Booth, M., *Opium, A History* (London, 1996).

Bowman, W.C., *A Dictionary of Pharmacology* (London, 1986).

Box, S., *Deviance, Reality and Society* (London, 1981).

Brookner, A., *Romanticism and its Discontents* (London, 2000).

Brown, G.H., ed., *Munk's Roll. Lives of the Fellows of the Royal College of Physicians of London, 1826-1925* (London, 1955).

Brown, L., *Victorian News and Newspapers* (OUP, 1985).

Burnett, J., *Plenty and Want: A Social History of Diet in England from 1815 to the Present Day* (London, 1966).

Butler, M., *Romantics, Rebels, and Reactionaries: English literature and its background, 1760-1830* (OUP, 1981).

Butts, J.S., *British MS Diaries of the Nineteenth Century: An annotated listing* (London, 1976).

Bynum, W.F., and Porter, R., eds, *Medical Fringe and Medical Orthodoxy, 1750-1850* (London, 1987).

———, Locke, S.,and Porter, R., eds, *Medical Journals and Medical Knowledge: Historical Essays* (London, 1992).

Checkland, S.G., *The Gladstones* (London, 1974).

Christison, *The Life of Sir Robert Christison*, BART., 2 vols (London, 1935).

Clarke, W.M., *The Secret Life of Wilkie Collins* (London, 1988).

Coomber, R., ed., *Drugs and Drug Use in Society: A critical reader* (Greenwich University Press, 1994).

Coombs, H. and P., *Journal of a Somerset Rector, 1803-1834* (OUP, 1984).

Daly, G., *Pre-Raphaelites in Lov*e (London, 1989).

De Almeida, H., *Romantic Medicine and John Keats* (OUP, 1991).

Douglas, M., *Purity and Danger: An analysis of the concept of pollution and taboo* (London, 1966).

Du Maurier, D., *The Infernal World of Branwell Brontë* (London, 1960).

Eaton, H.A., *Thomas De Quincey: A Biography* (London, 1936).

Ellman, R., *Oscar Wilde* (London, 1987).

Faden, A.I., and Sharpe, V.A., *Medical Harm: Historical, Conceptual, and Ethical Dimensions of Iatrogenic Illness* (CUP, 1998).

Fleck, L., *Genesis and Development of a Scientific Fact* (1935; edited and adapted by Trenn, T.J. and Merton, R.K. (London, 1979).

Flint, K., ed., *The Victorian Novelist: Social Problems and Social Change* (London, 1987).

Ford, J., *Coleridge on Dreaming: Romanticism and the Medical Imagination* (CUP, 1998).

Frank, L., *Charles Dickens and the Romantic Self* (University of Nebraska Press, 1984).

French, R., and Weir, A., eds, *British Medicine in an Age of Reform* (London, 1991).

Gagnier, R., *Subjectivities: A History of Self-Representation in Britain, 1832-1920* (OUP, 1991).

Gay, P., *The Bourgeois Experience, Victoria to Freud* (OUP, 1984).

———, *The Cultivation of Hatred* (London, 1994).

———, *The Naked Heart* (London, 1995).

———, *The Pleasure Wars* (London, 1998).

Gibson Lockhart, J., *The Life of Sir Walter Scott*, vol.6 (Edinburgh, 1902).

Gissing, G., *Forster's Life of Dickens* (London, 1903).

Glendinning, V., *Anthony Trollope* (London, 1993).

Golby, J.M., *Culture and Society in Britain, 1850-1890* (OUP, 1986).

Goodman, L.S., and Gillman, A.F., *The Pharmacological Basis of Therapeutics* (NY, 1996).

Gosling, F.G., *Before Freud: Neurasthenia and the American Medical Community, 1870-1910* (Cornell University Press, 1987).

Gould, A., *A History of Hypnotism* (CUP, 1992).

Griggs, E.L., ed., *The Collected Letters of Samuel Taylor Coleridge*, 6 vols (OUP, 1956-71).

Grinstein, A., *Freud at the Crossroads* (London, 1990).

Hale, N.G., *Freud in America: The beginnings of psychoanalysis in the United States, 1876-1917* (OUP, 1971).

Hampden, J., and Valance, R., *Charles Lamb: Essays* (London, 1963).

Harding, G., *Opiate Addiction, Morality and Medicine: from moral illness to pathological disease* (London, 1988).

Harrison, B., *Drink and the Victorians: The Temperance Question in England, 1815-1872* (Keele University Press, 1971).

Hawkins, J., *The Life of Samuel Johnson* (London, 1962).

Hayter, A., *Opium and the Romantic Imagination: addiction and creativity in De Quincey, Coleridge, Baudelaire and others* (London, 1968).

Henderson, A.K., *Romantic Identities: Varieties of Subjectivity, 1774-1830* (CUP, 1996).

Hilton, B., *The Age of Atonement: The influence of evangelicalism on social and economic thought, 1785-1865* (Oxford, 1988).

Hine, R.L., *Charles Lamb and his Hertfordshire* (London, 1949).

Hodge, B., *Opium: A portrait of the heavenly demon* (London, 2000).

Hogg, J., *De Quincey and his Friends* (London, 1895).

Holmes, R., *Shelley: The Pursuit* (London, 1994).

———, *Coleridge* (London, 1982).

———, *Coleridge: Early Visions* (London, 1989).

———, *Coleridge: Darker Reflections* (London, 1998).

Houghton, W.E., *The Victorian Frame of Mind 1830-1870* (Yale University Press, 1963).

Howe, W.D., *Charles Lamb and his Friends* (London, 1944).

Jackson, H.J., ed., *Samuel Taylor Coleridge: Selected Letters* (Oxford, 1987).

Jalland, P., *Death in the Victorian Family* (OUP, 1996).

Jay, M., *Emperors of Dreams: Drugs in the Nineteenth Century* (Cambridge, 2000).

Jones, K., *A Passionate Sisterhood: the sisters, wives, and daughters of the Lake Poets* (London, 1997).

Kiple, K.F., ed., *The Cambridge World History of Human Disease* (CUP, 1993).

Kuhn, T.S., *Structure of Scientific Revolutions* (Chicago, 1970).

Lambert, S., ed., *House of Commons Sessional Papers* (London, 1975) pp.219-26.

Landis, R., and Freeman, R., *Letters of the Brownings to George Barrett* (Illinois, 1958).

Latour, B., *Science in Action: how to follow scientists and engineers through society* (Harvard University Press, 1987).

Leask, N., *British Romantic Writers and the East: Anxieties of Empire* (CUP, 1993).

Lefebure, M., *Coleridge: A Bondage of Opium* (London, 1974).

Levine, S.M., *The Romantic Art of Confession* (London, 1998).

Lindesmith, A.R., and Strauss, A.L., eds, *Readings in Social Psychology* (London, 1969).

Lindop, G., *The Opium-Eater: A Life of Thomas De Quincey* (London, 1981).

Litchfield, R.B., *Tom Wedgewood: The First Photographer* (London, 1903).

Logan, P.M., *Nerves and Narratives: a cultural history of hysteria in nineteenth-century British prose* (London, 1997).

Lutz, T., *American Nervousness, 1903: an anecdotal history* (Cornell University Press, 1991).

McLaren, A., *A Prescription for Murder: the Victorian serial killings of Dr. Thomas Neill Cream* (London, 1993).

Markus, J., *Dared and Done: the marriage of Elizabeth Barrett and Robert Browning* (London, 1995).

Masson, D., *The Collected Writings of Thomas De Quincey* (Edinburgh, 1889-90).

Micale, M.S., *Approaching Hysteria: disease and its interpretations* (Princeton University Press, 1995).

Mikhail, E.H., *Oscar Wilde: Interviews and Recollections*, vol.1 (London, 1979).

Milligan, B., *Pleasures and Pains: Opium and the Orient in Nineteenth-Century British Culture* (University Press of Virginia, 1995).

Monk, W., ed., *The Journals of Caroline Fox, 1835-1871* (London, 1972).

Oppenheim, J., *"Shattered Nerves": Doctors, Patients, and Depression in Victorian England* (OUP, 1991).

Parssinen, T.M., *Secret Passions, Secret Remedies: Narcotic Drugs in British Society, 1820-1930* (Manchester, 1983).

Pasternak, G.W., *The Opiate Receptors* (New Jersey, 1988).

Pearsall, R., *Conan Doyle: A Biographical Solution* (Glasgow, 1977).

Peele, S., *The Meaning of Addiction: Compulsive experience and its interpretation* (Massachusetts, 1985).

———, ed., *Visions of Addiction: Major contemporary perspectives on addiction and alcoholism* (Massachusetts, 1988).

Phillips, A., *Charles Lamb: selected prose* (London, 1985).

Pick, D., *Faces of Degeneration: A European Disorder, c.1848-c.1918* (CUP, 1989).

Pickering, G., *Creative Malady: illness in the lives of Charles Darwin, Florence Nightingale, Mary Baker Eddy, Sigmund Freud, Marcel Proust, Elizabeth Barrett Browning* (London, 1974).

Pollock, J., *William Wilberforce* (London, 1977).

Porter, R., *Mind-Forg'd Manacles: a history of madness in England from the Restoration to the Regency* (London, 1987).

———, *The Cambridge Illustrated History of Medicine* (CUP, 1996).

———, *The Great Benefit to Mankind: a medical history of humanity from antiquity to the present* (London, 1997).

———, and Rousseau, G.S., eds, *Sexual Underworlds of the Enlightenment* (Manchester University Press, 1987).

———, and Teich, M., eds, *Drugs and Narcotics in History* (CUP, 1995).

———, and Teich, M., eds, *Sexual Knowledge and Sexual Science: the history of attitudes to sexual knowledge* (CUP, 1994).

Prioreschi, P., *A History of Medicine* (Omaha, 1998).

Proudfoot, A.T., *Acute Poisoning: Diagnosis and Management* (Oxford, 1993).

Richardson, R., *Death, Dissection, and the Destitute* (London, 1988).

Rose, L., *Massacre of the Innocents: infanticide in Great Britain, 1800-1939* (London, 1986).

Rudgley, R., *An Anthology of Wildest Dreams: Drug Related Literature* (London, 1999).

Schaffer, H., and Burglass, M.E., eds, *Classic Contributions to the Addictions* (London, 1981).

Scull, A., *Museums of Madness: The Social Organization of Insanity in Nineteenth-Century England* (London, 1979).

———, *The Most Solitary of Afflictions: Madness and Society in Britain 1700-1900* (London, 1993).

Segen, J., *Current Medical Talk: A Dictionary of Medical Terms, Slang, and Jargon* (Connecticut, 1995).

Shorter, E., *From Paralysis to Fatigue: A History of Psychosomatic Illness in the Modern Era* (London, 1992).
Sills, D.L., ed., *International Encyclopaedia of the Social Sciences* (NY, 1968).
Silverstone, T., and Turner, P., *Drug Treatment in Psychiatry* (London, 1978).
Skinner, H., *The Origin of Medical Terms* (NY, 1970).
Skinner, J., *Journal of a Somerset Rector, 1803-1834* (London, 1930).
Smith, F.B., *The People's Health, 1830-1910* (London, 1979).
Sontag, S., *Illness as Metaphor* (London, 1979).
Sournia, J-C., *A History of Alcoholism* (Oxford, 1990).
South, N., *Drugs, Crime, and Criminal Justice*, 2 vols (Dartmouth, 1995).
Spillane, J.D., *The Doctrine of the Nerves: Chapters in the History of Neurology* (OUP, 1981).
Steib, E.W., *Drug Adulteration: Detection and Control in Nineteenth-Century Britain* (Wisconsin, 1966).
Stone, D.D., *The Romantic Impulse in Victorian Fiction* (London, 1980).
Strausbaugh, J., and Blaise, D., eds, *The Drug Use Documents, 1840-1960* (NY, 1990).
Symons, J., *Portrait of an Artist: Conan Doyle* (London, 1979).
Szasz, T., *Ceremonial Chemistry: The ritual persecution of drugs, addicts, and pushers* (London, 1974).
Turner, J., *Herbert Spencer: A Renewed Appreciation* (London, 1985).
Veith, I., *Hysteria: The History of a Disease* (Chicago, 1965).
Vickers, N., *Coleridge and the Doctors 1795-1806* (OUP, 2004).
Walton, J., Beeson, P., and Bodley Scott, R., eds, *The Oxford Companion to Medicine*, 2 vols (OUP, 1986).
Wear, A., *Medicine in Society: Historical Essays* (CUP, 1992).
Weeks, J., *Sex, Politics and Society: The regulation of sexuality since 1800* (London, 1989).
Weissman, S., *His Brother's Keeper: A Psychobiography of Samuel Taylor Coleridge* (Connecticut, 1989).
Westermeyer, J., *Poppies, Pipes, and People: Opium and its Use in Laos* (California, 1982).
Williams, N., *Contraband Cargoes: Seven Centuries of Smuggling* (London, 1959).

Dissertations

Turner, T, 'A diagnostic analysis of the casebooks of Ticehurst House Asylum', Unpublished MD thesis (London, 1991).

Articles

Bartrip, P., 'A "Pennurth of arsenic for rat poison": the Arsenic Act, 1851, and the prevention of secret poisoning', *Medical History* (1992) 36, pp.53-69.
Berridge, V., 'Opium and the historical perspective', *Lancet* (1977) 2, pp.78-80.

———, 'Opium eating and life insurance', *British Journal of Addiction* (1977) 72, pp.371-7

———,'East End opium dens and narcotic use in Britain', *London Journal* (1978) 4, pp.3-28.

———,'Victorian opium eating: responses to opiate use in nineteenth-century society', *Victorian Studies* (1978) 4, pp.437-61.

———,'Opium over the counter in nineteenth-century England', *Pharmacy in History* (1978) 3, pp.91-100.

———,'Opium and oral history', *Journal of Oral history* (1979) 7, pp.48-58.

Burney, I.A., 'A poisoning of no substance: the trials of medico-legal proof in mid-Victorian Britain', *Journal of British Studies* (1999) 38, pp.59-92.

Bynum, W.F., 'Chronic alcoholism in the first half of the nineteenth century, *Bulletin of the History of Medicine* (1968) xlii, pp.160-85.

Carlson, E.T., 'George M. Beard and Neurasthenia', in *Essays in the History of Psychiatry*, 10th anniversary supplementary volume to *Psychiatric Forum*, Wallace, E., and Pressley, L., NY (1980) pp.50-7.

Clarke, M.J., 'Suicides by opium and its derivatives in England and Wales, 1850-1950', *Psychological Medicine* (1985) 15, pp.237-42.

Collins, P., 'Inspector Bucket visits the Princess Puffer', *The Dickensian* (1964) 60, pp.88-90.

Edwards, G., 'Opium and after', *Lancet* (1980) 1, pp.351-4.

Hardcastle, V.G., 'What we don't know about brains', *Studies in the History and Philosophy of Biological and Biomedical Sciences* (1999) 30C, pp.69-90.

Harris, M., 'Social diseases? Crime and medicine in the Victorian press', in Bynum, Locke and Porter, *Medical Journals and Medical Knowledge* (1992) pp.108-25.

Howard-Jones, N., 'Critical study of the origins and early development of hypodermic medication', *Journal of the History of Medicine*, Spring (1947) pp.201-47.

Macht, D.I., and Gessford, N.L., 'The unfortunate drug experiences of Dante Gabriel Rossetti', *Institute of the History of Medicine Bulletin* (1938) 6, pp.34-61.

McLeod, R., 'The edge of hope: social policy and chronic alcoholism, 1870-1900', *Journal of the History of Medicine*, July (1967) pp.215-45.

Morris, A.R., 'Oscar Wilde and the eclipse of Darwinism: aestheticism, degeneration, and moral reaction in late-Victorian ideology', *Studies in the History and Philosophy of Science* (1993) 24, pp.513-40.

Moss, G.L., 'Masculinity and Decadence', in Porter and Teich, *Sexual Knowledge and Sexual Science*, (1994) pp. 251-66.

O'Malley, P., and Mugford, S., 'The demand for intoxicating commodities: implications for the "War on Drugs"', *Social Justice* (1988) 18, pp.49-75.

Parssinen, T., 'Essay review of Berridge and Edwards, *Opium*', *Medical History* (1982) pp.458-62.

———, and Kerner, K., 'The development of the disease model of addiction in Britain, 1870-1926', *Medical History* (1980) 24, pp.275-96.

Porter, I.A., 'Thomas Trotter, MD., Naval Physician', *Medical History* (1963) 7, pp.155-64.

Porter, R., 'The drinking man's disease: the pre-history of alcoholism in Georgian Britain', *British Journal of Addiction* (1985) 80, pp.385-96.

Pruitt, A., 'Approaches to alcoholism in mid-Victorian Britain', *Clio Medica* (1974) 9, pp.93-101.

Sonnedecker, G., 'Emergence of the concept of opiate addiction', *Journal Mondial de Pharmacie* (1962) 3, pp.275-90.

For modern works that shed light on the international aspect of opiate addiction, see the following:

Courtwright, D., *Dark Paradise. Opiate Addiction in America before 1940* (London, 1982).

Goodman, J., Lovejoy, P.E., and Sherrat, A., eds, *Consuming Habits. Drugs in History and Anthropology* (London, 1995).

Kohn, M., *Narcomania* (London, 1987).

Kramer, J.C., 'Opium Rampant: Medical Use, Misuse and Abuse in Britain and the West in the Seventeenth and Eighteenth Centuries', *British Journal of Addiction* (1979) 74, pp.377-89.

———, 'The Opiates: Two Centuries of Scientific Study', *Journal of Psychedelic Drugs* (1980) 12, pp.89-103.

Musto, D.F., *The American Disease. Origins of Narcotic Control* (OUP, 1999).

Terry, C.E., & Pellens, M., *The Opium Problem* (NY, 1928).

Index

B

M

N

O

S

T

U

V

W

Y

Z